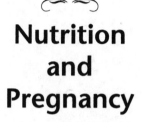

Nutrition
and
Pregnancy

Nutrition
and
Pregnancy

*A Complete Guide
from Preconception to Postdelivery*

by
JUDITH E. BROWN, R.D., M.P.H., PH.D.

Foreword by
HOWARD N. JACOBSON, M.D.

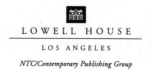

LOWELL HOUSE

LOS ANGELES

NTC/Contemporary Publishing Group

"Recipes for Healthy Eating" are reprinted with permission by Margaret Reinhardt, M.P.H., licensed nutritionist, and Barbara Turgeon, certified home economist. Copyright © 1988 Nutrition Plus, Inc., Minneapolis, Minnesota.

This book is in no way intended to replace the advice of a physician. All matters regarding your health require medical supervision.

Library of Congress Cataloging in Publication Data
Brown, Judith E.
    Nutrition and pregnancy : a complete guide from preconception to post-delivery / by Judith E. Brown ; foreword by Howard N. Jacobson.
        p.   cm.
    Includes bibliographical references and index.
    ISBN 1-56565-790-X (hardcover)
    ISBN 0-7373-0018-3 (paperback)
    1. Pregnancy—Nutritional aspects. I. Title.
RG559.B758   1998
618.2'4—dc21   97-38624
                                                                           CIP

Requests for such permissions should be addressed to:
Lowell House
2020 Avenue of the Stars, Suite 300
Los Angeles, CA   90067

Published by Lowell House, a division of NTC/Contemporary Publishing Group, Inc.
4255 West Touhy Avenue, Lincolnwood, Illinois 60646-1975 U.S.A.

Design by Andrea Reider

Printed and bound in the United States of America
International Standard Book Number: 0-7373-0018-3
    8 9 10 DOC/DOC 0 9 8 7 6 5 4

Behind every advance in knowledge that leads to improvements in quality of life are individuals who, without benefit to themselves, volunteer to take part in research studies. Here's to the women who participate in research that advances our knowledge about nutrition and fertility, pregnancy, and breast-feeding. You benefit our children and all of us. This book is dedicated to you.

Acknowledgments

I feel a deep indebtedness to those who have directed my interest toward producing that ounce of prevention worth a pound of cure. My daughter Amanda and my son Max piqued my interest in this area. I have learned many lessons about the nutritional ounce of prevention from Agnes Higgins, the former director of the Montreal Diet Dispensary; Howard Jacobson and Charles Mahan, obstetricians who promote prevention; and Sally Lederman of Columbia University, who is a crystal-clear thinker about evidence related to nutrition and pregnancy outcome. I have been given the opportunity to learn about nutrition and pregnancy and to write and teach about what I learned by grants from the National Institute of Child Health and Human Development and the Maternal and Child Health Bureau of the Public Health Service. My primary instructors, however, have been and will remain those wonderful women who volunteer to participate in research studies.

Contents

⌒ Preface ⌒

Looking for information about preparing your body for pregnancy? Is it taking longer than you had hoped to become pregnant? Are you pregnant and concerned that you may be gaining too much weight, or unsure about which foods and supplements you should consume and which you should avoid? Do you need to know about nutrition for twin pregnancy? Are you anticipating a need for facts about breast-feeding or getting your body back into shape after your baby is born? If questions and concerns like these brought you to the bookstore or library, you have found the right book.

Chapter 1 begins with an overview of the benefits of good nutrition for pregnancy. Chapter 2 provides basic information on nutrition, including facts about vitamins and minerals and their leading food sources. Specific nutrition tables presented in Chapter 2 are referred to often throughout the book.

Pregnancy begins with conception, but conception may be the weak link. Chapter 3 addresses the role of nutrition in fertility and how changes in nutritional status can affect your chances of becoming pregnant. Many conditions affect fertility, and scientists have much more to learn about why some women conceive right away while others may never become pregnant.

Perhaps the greatest advances in our knowledge about nutrition and pregnancy in the past ten years have been made in the area of preconceptional and early pregnancy nutrition. Chapter 4 highlights these advances and gives specific recommendations on optimal nutrition for early fetal development and growth. This chapter provides instructions on how to evaluate your current diet and what you can do to improve it.

Chapter 5 describes "the right diet for pregnancy" and answers frequently asked questions about diet during this time. The pros and cons of using vitamin and mineral supplements during pregnancy and indications for their use are covered in Chapter 6.

How much and when a woman gains weight during pregnancy have important influences on fetal growth and development. Chapter 7 includes a weight-gain graph that can be used to monitor progress. Closely aligned with weight gain is the topic of exercise, so Chapter 8 explains the whys and hows of exercising during pregnancy.

Pregnancy has a number of "side effects" that would be considered abnormal in women who are not pregnant. These common and bothersome problems can sometimes be effectively prevented or managed with changes in diet, exercise, or the use of supplements. Chapter 9 covers nutritional aids for nausea and vomiting, heartburn, and constipation. Background information on and nutritional recommendations for conditions that arise during pregnancy, such as gestational diabetes, preeclampsia, and iron deficiency anemia, are also covered in this chapter.

What nutritional guidance is available for women pregnant with twins? Nutritional recommendations for women "eating for three" are covered in Chapter 10. Notes to women bearing triplets are also given, but this information is quite tentative since appropriate studies are yet to be done. The final two chapters address postpregnancy topics. Chapter 11 includes infant nutrition and feeding recommendations; Chapter 12 is devoted to the topic of breast-feeding.

I encourage readers to peruse Appendix A. The recipes for healthy eating at the back of this book have been designed and tested by a nutritionist and a home economist and include nutritional information.

Literally thousands of research reports and other sources of dependable information about nutrition and fertility, pregnancy, and breast-feeding were used during the development of this book. Because space considerations preclude listing them all, only key references and those to which women may wish to refer for additional information are included.

Throughout this book women are referred to as the primary audience. This is because women are in the best position to act upon the information. Clearly, spouses, partners, in-laws, and grandparents-to-be may be interested in these topics and provide much valued support. Reference to women is not meant to exclude other interested or involved individuals.

Nutrition and Pregnancy has been developed using state-of-the-art information. Only scientifically supported recommendations related to nutrition and reproduction are included in this book. However, knowledge about maternal nutrition is continuously expanding, and new, important developments may not be addressed here. For this reason, and because they may affect the type of health care you receive, you are urged to keep your health care provider informed about your concerns and actions related to diet, supplement use, and weight.

Best wishes for good humor, happiness, and a bundle of joy,

JUDITH E. BROWN

⊂ Foreword ⊃

Pregnant women have always accepted the importance of good nutrition, and health professionals are finally realizing just how important it is for pregnancy, as well as fertility and breast-feeding. In the last ten years there has been a veritable explosion of books, pamphlets, and guides for pregnant women. In most cases, information prepared by professionals was either too technical or too impersonal for the general public. At the other extreme, popular books prepared for the layperson have tended to lack enough scientific credibility.

In *Nutrition and Pregnancy,* Judith Brown fulfills her intention of writing a readable, useful, and accurate guide that is both upbeat and supportive in tone. Essential topics are covered with sufficient detail, helping women make the right choices about diet, supplement use, weight gain, and infant feeding.

With its combination of impeccable accuracy and positive emphasis, this book will be a major influence in helping women become nutritionally prepared for conception, pregnancy, and breast-feeding.

HOWARD N. JACOBSON, M.D.
Professor, Dept. of Community and Family Health,
College of Public Health, University of South Florida

Nutrition
and
Pregnancy

Giving Yourself and Your Baby the Nutritional Advantage

The conception and the delivery of a healthy baby are influenced by many conditions that are both within and outside of our control. Of those within our control, nutrition is primary. The type of diet a woman consumes before and during pregnancy can influence fertility and pregnancy in multiple ways. Under the right circumstances, good nutrition can be a gift, an above-average start on life and health advantages that last for a lifetime.

Today we are experiencing an explosion in new information about nutrition and fertility, pregnancy, and breast-feeding. A renaissance in research is underway, and it is redefining what nutritional advice should be given to women who are attempting to conceive or who are pregnant or breast-feeding. Advice previously based on clinical assumptions or personal biases is being replaced with recommendations supported by solid evidence. There are important advantages to the scientifically supported recommendations that are emerging from today's studies: They have been demonstrated to benefit health and they hold up over time.

Out with the Old Advice

It wasn't that long ago when nutritional factors were regarded as being unrelated to fertility. We now know that body weight, location of body fat stores, usual diet, and supplement use all influence fertility. It used to be thought that the fetus was a parasite, extracting from the mother whatever nutrients it needed for growth and development regardless of the mother's diet. (Some people still believe this is true today.) It is now commonly accepted that the fetus is not a parasite; it does not benefit while harming the mother. The nourishment of the fetus depends on the supply of nutrients from the mother's diet and her nutrient stores. In order to ensure survival of the species, it is the mother who gets primary access to most nutrients if nutrient supply is low. A healthy mother can reproduce again.

In the past, women were said to have maternal instincts that would direct them to select and consume nutritious foods during pregnancy. This notion is as valid as the ancient Roman belief that if you wanted a child with dark eyes you should eat mice often. Other common ideas such as the recommendation that all women should take multivitamins and mineral supplements, restrict their salt intake, and diet to keep their weight low in pregnancy are no longer supported.

New information about nutrition and fertility, pregnancy, and infant feeding emerges constantly, and it is difficult for health care providers to stay current on all the advances. Unfortunately, many providers are not up-to-date on the low-tech, nondrug nutritional improvements that could benefit the women they serve.

In with the New

Much of the earlier advice given to women about nutrition and reproduction was insufficiently supported by scientific research and heavily biased by unproven assumptions. As knowledge expands, so should the specific recommendations given to women about nutrition. Some advances in nutrition information slowly seep into health care; others seem to be kept secret. A number of nutritional measures can be undertaken to enhance the chances of conception for many women. It is also clear that a growing and developing fetus is vulnerable to the influence of energy and nutrients it receives from the mother, and that excessive vitamins and minerals from supplements may be as hazardous to fetal well-being as deficient amounts. It is now known that a woman's intake of certain vitamins, such as folate, vitamin A, and vitamin D, very early in pregnancy can be related to the development of certain malformations in the baby. How much weight women gain in pregnancy, and the timing of the gain, have important effects on the risk of preterm delivery and the size and health status of infants at birth.

One of the most striking advances in research concerns maternal nutrition and the subsequent risk of certain chronic diseases. It appears that a predisposition for heart disease, diabetes, high blood pressure, and a number of other diseases and disorders may be "programmed" by inadequate supplies of energy or nutrients during pregnancy and early infancy. A large body of evidence indicates that newborns with optimal growth may be at lower risk for developing these health problems later in life.

Well-nourished women are also less likely to experience miscarriages, or to develop iron deficiency anemia, constipation, fatigue, and other common problems of pregnancy. Babies born to well-nourished women are more likely to be born in robust health, to feed vigorously, to grow optimally, and to be alert and responsive. Although there is much more to be learned about the effects of nutrition on fetal growth, development, and subsequent health, the influence of maternal nutrition is being recognized, and the advantages of optimal nutrition are more extensive than previously imagined.

Good News

One of the best things about nutrition is that the risks associated with poor eating habits can often be eliminated by fixing the weak link in nutritional health. It may be as simple as consuming more of your favorite fruits and vegetables, eating a breakfast cereal fortified with folic acid, or taking a low-dose iron supplement. Some steps may be more difficult, such as gaining weight or cutting down on some of your favorite junk foods. But these gifts you give to your unborn baby will benefit you as well. Your reward may be a perfectly timed conception, higher energy levels during pregnancy, less intense side effects of pregnancy (such as nausea and vomiting, constipation, and heartburn), or a fully grown and developed newborn that is easy to care for.

Despite the best efforts, not everyone who wants to become pregnant will, and not all pregnancies will end in healthy newborns. Although it is very important, nutrition is not the only factor that influences fertility or pregnancy. Problems arise due to a myriad of factors that can be identified but not always remedied. In addition, there are probably hundreds of causes of infertility and pregnancy problems that have yet to be identified. These many unknowns make it impossible to chart a course that guarantees conception and a healthy newborn. With so many mysteries, blaming oneself for problems of uncertain origin is unreasonable and should be resisted with all the strength the spirit can muster. Keeping this in mind, the best course to chart is one that is within your control. The specific information you need to follow the right nutrition path will be provided to you in the upcoming chapters.

⮑ 2 ⮐

The Truth About Nutrition and Healthy Diets

Welcome to Nutrition 101: A crash course on how substances in foods affect health. Unlike a typical college course, the contents are condensed, and there are no tuition costs, pop quizzes, or papers due. It is included in this book to provide you good general background information about nutrition, and which will help you make the right decisions about your diet. Use this chapter to learn as much, or as little, as you want or need, and remember it's here if you need to look up a fact or to check out something you read or hear about nutrition.

This chapter presents core knowledge, or principles, upon which the science of nutrition is based. Included within the discussion are ways this knowledge can be personally applied to promote health before, during, and after pregnancy. Subsequent chapters address the application of nutrition knowledge to fertility, pregnancy, infant feeding, and breast-feeding. In this chapter you will find information on nutrients and other substances in foods that benefit health, recommended levels of nutrient intake, vegetarianism, and how to obtain a healthy diet. The final section of the chapter provides a prescription for diagnosing the truthfulness of nutrition information presented to consumers. Without some guidelines, it can be very difficult to determine if what you hear or read about nutrition is fact or fantasy.

Nutrition Principles

The basic truths about nutrition can be summarized in seven principles. These principles change little with time and serve as the foundation for growth in knowledge about nutrition and health.

1. Food Is a Basic Need of Humans

The first nutrition principle is straightforward. Humans need food to grow, to reproduce, and to stay healthy. Food also represents one of the greatest pleasures on Earth. It provides relief from hunger and a feeling of comfort and security. Beyond survival, food is basic to a full and healthy life.

2. Humans Require Nutrients Found in Foods for Growth, Reproduction, and Health

The need for food is based on the body's requirement for nutrients, or specific chemical substances in food that perform particular functions in the body. There are only six categories of nutrients:

1. carbohydrates
2. proteins
3. fats
4. vitamins
5. minerals
6. water

Carbohydrates, proteins, and fats supply calories and are called the "energy nutrients." Although these three types of nutrients perform a variety of functions, they share the property of being the body's source of energy. Vitamins, minerals, and water are primarily needed for the conversion of carbohydrates, proteins, and fats into energy, and for the building and maintenance of muscles, blood components, bones, and other body parts. Water serves as a medium for most chemical reactions that take place in the body, it is needed for the removal of waste products in urine, and it functions as the body's cooling system.

The Energy Nutrients

The first and foremost need of the body is for energy, or the *calories* supplied by food. Calories are not a component of food. Rather, they represent the amount of energy supplied by the carbohydrate, protein, and fat content of foods. Most carbohydrates and proteins supply 4 calories per gram, while fat provides over twice that much—9 calories per gram. (There are 28 grams in 1 ounce; 1 ounce is 2 tablespoons of liquid.) If you have observed the flames produced by dripping fat from a steak or hamburger on a grill, you have seen the powerhouse of energy stored in fat. Foods high in carbohydrates or protein, such as corn, potatoes, fish, or shrimp, don't burn with nearly the same intensity when grilled. They have less energy to give. Alcohol, a fermentation product of carbohydrates, provides 7 calories per gram. The relatively high energy content of alcohol makes the preparation of cherries jubilee and crepes suzette possible.

When we consume more calories from food than our bodies need, the excess is largely converted to fat and stored for later use. The body is not picky. It converts excessive incoming supplies of carbohydrates, fats, and proteins into storage fat. Carbohydrates can also be stored in the body in the form of glycogen. However, glycogen stores are much smaller than our fat stores. People are usually limited to about an 1,800-calorie supply of glycogen stored in muscles and the liver. The human ability to store fat, on the other hand, can be extraordinary and averages about 140,000 calories in adults. When fewer calories are taken in than needed, we draw upon our energy stores, reducing both them and our overall weight.

There is much more to learn about the energy nutrients. This information is condensed into the highlights that follow.

Carbohydrates

Carbohydrates are the world's leading source of human energy. Foods rich in carbohydrates, such as rice, potatoes, dried beans, millet, cassava, pasta, and breads, are the main ingredients of people's diets throughout most of the world. The United States and several other economically developed countries stand out from the rest of the world in that carbohydrates take a back seat to foods rich in protein and fat.

Many different substances in foods are classified as carbohydrates. The two major types are the *simple sugars* and the *complex carbohydrates*. Alcohol, because it formed from carbohydrates, is categorized as a carbohydratelike substance.

The simple sugars. There are three major sugars that are as simple as carbohydrates get: glucose (blood sugar), fructose (fruit sugar), and galactose (milk sugar). Nearly all of the fructose and galactose consumed in foods is rapidly converted to glucose by the body. Glucose is the only form of sugar that can be used by the body to make energy.

Simple sugars come in packages of two units of glucose, fructose, and/or galactose. Maltose (malt sugar) consists of two units of glucose, whereas sucrose, or table sugar, and honey are formed from glucose and fructose. The milk sugar fructose contains glucose plus galactose.

Most of the simple sugars have a very distinctive sweet taste, which is why many people love to eat them. Humans, like most mammals, are born with a preference for sweet-tasting foods. Even before birth, a fetus will move toward a sucrose solution injected into the womb. It will withdraw from bitter and sour-tasting fluids. After birth, infants will select sweet-tasting liquids over those with other flavors. Interestingly, breast milk tastes sweet.

Most of the simple sugars in the American diet are added to foods before purchase. Of the total amount of sugar produced, about 65 percent is used by the food and beverage industry and the manufacturers of soft drinks, beer, wine, bakery products, cereals, candy, and processed foods. One 12-ounce cola, for example, contains about 8 teaspoons of sugar. Some presweetened cereals have 4 teaspoons of added sugar per serving. Added sugars can make up as much as 45 percent of the total calories in breakfast cereal. You can find out how much sugar is in a breakfast cereal, and in many other foods, by checking the nutrition information panel on the package.

Is there good reason to swallow a side order of guilt along with your favorite treats? Do sweets deserve their reputation as being bad for you? Do they cause hyperactivity, diabetes, obesity, and tooth decay?

Sugars, by themselves, are not bad for you nor are they responsible for hyperactivity in children, diabetes, or obesity. It is true that frequent snacking on sweet foods, and a failure to clean your teeth after consuming sticky sweets, can lead to tooth decay. This is much more likely to occur in people whose local water supply is not fluoridated.

There is another problem related to sugars that depends on the quantity of sugary foods consumed. Goodies like candy, sherbet, soft drinks, and cookies are usually a poor source of vitamins, minerals, and other beneficial components of food. If too many sweet foods are eaten, they replace other, more nutrient-dense foods in the diet, such as vegetables, fruits, and whole-grain products. Large intakes of sweet foods may contribute to excessively high caloric consumption and to disorders such as adult-onset diabetes (Type II diabetes), hypertension, and heart disease, which are related to being overweight. No more than 10 percent of your total calorie intake should come from simple sugars.

The complex carbohydrates. The complex carbohydrates consist of *starches, glycogen,* and *dietary fiber* (or "bulk"). Complex carbohydrates come to us from plants and, although many are formed by combinations of glucose units, they all lack the sweet taste of simple sugars. Because animal products contain very little glycogen, almost all of the starch in our diets comes from plants such as dried beans, potatoes, corn, wheat, and rice. These plants store glucose as starch. Starch consumed in the diet is broken down by digestive enzymes into glucose. Food sources of starch are not only high in glucose, but they provide vitamins, minerals, dietary fiber, and other elements required for health.

Recommendations for health-promoting diets indicate that 50 to 60 percent of our total calories should come from carbohydrates, particularly food sources of the complex carbohydrates (see Table 2–1).

Dietary fiber. Dietary fiber differs from starches in that it is not digested by enzymes produced by humans. Consequently, it is not considered to be a source of energy.

Dietary fiber is found only in plants and comes in two basic types. One type is the fibrous components of plant cells, particularly plant cell walls. The other type is nonfibrous components of plant cells that are primarily found inside of cells. Dietary fiber, even though it is not absorbed into the body proper, has a number of effects. The specific effect varies according to what type of dietary fiber is consumed. Fibrous forms of dietary fiber, such as that found

Table 2–1 Food Sources of Complex Carbohydrates

	Amount	Complex Carbohydrate (grams)	% of Total Calories from Complex Carbohydrates
Grain and Grain Products			
Rice	½ cup	21	83
Pasta	½ cup	15	81
Cornflakes	1 cup	11	76
Oatmeal	1½ cups	12	74
Cheerios	1 cup	11	68
Whole-wheat bread	1 slice	7	60
Dried Beans (cooked)			
Lima beans	½ cup	11	64
White beans	½ cup	13	63
Kidney beans	½ cup	12	59
Vegetables			
Carrot	1 medium	7	93
Potato	1 medium	30	85
Corn	½ cup	10	67
Broccoli	½ cup	2	40

in bran and fruit and vegetable skins, helps prevent constipation. Gel-forming nonfibrous fiber, such as that contained in the pulp of fruit, oatmeal, and dried beans, slows glucose absorption and decreases the amount of cholesterol that is absorbed from foods. This type of fiber also enhances elimination by forming bulk in the intestine that moves waste products along.

Many foods, such as dried beans, potatoes, and avocados, hide their high fiber content very well. They are not crunchy and don't look fibrous. Yet they are among our best sources of dietary fiber. Other foods that are crunchy, such as popcorn, lettuce, and celery, are not very high in fiber. The bottom line is that you can't tell a plant's fiber content by its looks or its crunch value. Table 2–2 shows the dietary fiber content of many foods and reveals the hidden truths.

Many people consume too little dietary fiber. Approximately 25 grams per day is thought to represent a healthful level of intake.

Table 2–2 Food Sources of Dietary Fiber

	Amount	Dietary Fiber (grams)
Grain and Cereal Products		
Bran Buds	1 cup	24
Bulgur, cooked	1 cup	11
All Bran	½ cup	10
40% Bran Flakes	1 cup	8
Bran muffin	1 large (4 ounces)	7
Cornmeal muffin	1 large (4 ounces)	7
Bran Chex	1 cup	7
Raisin Bran	1 cup	7
Bran	¼ cup	6
Grape-Nuts	¾ cup	6
Whole-wheat macaroni	1 cup	5
Shredded Wheat	1 biscuit	3
Oatmeal	¾ cup	2
Cornflakes	¾ cup	2
Whole-wheat bread	1 slice	2
Popcorn	2 cups	2
Fruits		
Avocado, mashed	1 cup	7
Raspberries	1 cup	5
Mango	1 medium	4
Pear (with skin)	1 medium	4
Strawberries	1 cup	4
Apple (with skin)	1 medium	3
Peach (with skin)	1 medium	3
Banana or plantain	6 inches long	2
Vegetables		
Corn, canned	½ cup	5
Lima beans	½ cup	5
Potato (with skin)	1 medium	3
Potato (no skin)	1 medium	2
Broccoli	½ cup	3
Carrots, boiled	½ cup	3
Green beans	½ cup	3
Brussels sprouts	½ cup	3
Eggplant	½ cup	3
Collard greens	½ cup	3

continued

Table 2–2 Food Sources of Dietary Fiber, *continued*

	Amount	Dietary Fiber (grams)
Nuts		
Almonds, Brazil nuts	1 ounce	3
Peanuts, pecans, macadamias	1 ounce	2
Peanut butter	2 tablespoons	2
Dried Beans		
Pinto beans	½ cup	10
Black beans	½ cup	8
White, kidney, navy beans	½ cup	7
Garbanzos (chickpeas)	½ cup	5
Lentils	½ cup	5
Peas	½ cup	4

Individuals vary in their ability to tolerate increased levels of dietary fiber. If you develop diarrhea after increasing your fiber intake, cut back. If constipation develops, drink more water.

Although human beings do not produce the types of digestive enzymes needed to break down dietary fiber, certain bacteria that dwell in the large intestines do. Bacteria that consume dietary fiber as food don't break down the fiber completely. They excrete fragments of fats and gases as end products of dietary fiber ingestion. Discomfort related to bacterial gas production with dietary fiber intake decreases over time.

Protein

There is little reason to write about the importance of protein; most people are already convinced of it. Protein is an essential structural component of all living matter. It is involved in most every biological process that takes place in humans. Although protein is used as an energy source, this is a secondary, rather than primary, role.

Proteins consist of units of amino acids linked together in chemical chains. It is really the amino acids that are needed for health, and not the protein per se. There are twenty amino acids that serve as building blocks for the thousands of proteins formed by the body.

Of these, nine are *essential,* meaning that they must be obtained through diet. The other eleven major amino acids are considered *nonessential* because they can be produced by the body. They still perform necessary roles in the body, however, and they are as important to health as the essential amino acids. They are only called nonessential because we don't have to obtain them from foods.

Proteins are classified by their ability to support protein tissue construction in the body. Not all sources of protein do this equally well; it depends on their content of essential amino acids. How well proteins in foods support the development and maintenance of protein tissues in the body is discovered by tests of the protein's *quality.*

Protein quality. Proteins are different from carbohydrates and fats in that they vary in quality. In general, animal products provide high-quality protein, and plant foods have lower protein quality. Unless proteins of high quality are eaten, people will not grow, reproduce, or stay healthy no matter how much protein is consumed.

High-quality proteins contain all the essential amino acids in the amounts needed to support protein tissue formation in the body. If any of the essential amino acids are lacking in dietary protein sources, protein tissues are not formed—even for those proteins that could be constructed from available amino acids. It may appear inefficient for the body to shut off protein tissue construction for the want of an amino acid or two. If protein tissue development did not shut down, however, cells would end up with an imbalanced assortment of protein that would seriously affect cell functions. Without the needed levels of each essential amino acid, proteins consumed can only be used to form energy.

Food sources of protein that contain all the essential amino acids in the amounts needed to support protein tissue construction are considered high quality or *complete proteins.* Proteins in this category include those found in animal products such as meat, milk, and eggs. *Incomplete proteins* are deficient in one or more amino acids. With the exception of soybean protein for adults, proteins found in plants are incomplete. However, you can complement the essential amino acids composition of plant sources by combining them to form a complete source of protein. Combining a grain such as rice, with a legume such as pinto beans provides a complete protein source. Complementary proteins can be obtained from plants by combining rice and green peas, bulgur and dried beans, barley and dried beans, corn and dried beans, corn and lima beans, and seeds and green peas.

Although it used to be thought that complementary proteins needed to be consumed at the same meal, this is no longer considered to be true. Combining vegetable sources of protein within the same day is adequate to obtain complete proteins.

Excessively restrictive or poorly planned vegetarian diets, especially when consumed by people with high nutrient needs such as women who are pregnant and children, can compromise health. Vegetarians need to take care to include food sources of iron, zinc, calcium, and vitamins B_{12} and D in their diets. Tables that list food sources of these nutrients are included in Appendix B.

Adult women require about 50 grams of protein a day and most American adults consume far more protein than required for health. You can estimate whether or not you are getting the right amount by examining Table 2–3.

Fats

Fats are a group of substances found in the body that have one major property in common: They dissolve in fat and not in water. If you have ever tried to get vinegar and oil to mix before you poured them over a salad, you have observed firsthand the principle of water and fat solubility.

Fats are actually a subcategory of the fat-soluble substances known as *lipids*. Lipids include all types of fats and oils. Fats are often distinguished from oils by their property of being solid at room temperature. Solid fat is generally high in saturated fat and of animal origin. Butter, lard, and animal fat belong in this group because they don't melt at room temperature. Oils, on the other hand, are liquid at room temperature. They contain primarily unsaturated fats from plants. A liquid oil can be changed to a solid fat by adding hydrogens, called hydrogenating the oil. Hydrogenated fats such as margarine and shortening still contain an abundance of unsaturated fats.

Table 2–3 Food Sources of Protein

Food	Amount	Protein Content grams	Protein Content % of total calories
Meat and Animal Products			
Cottage cheese, low-fat	1 cup	28	69
Pork chop, lean	3 ounces	27	36
Beef roast, lean	3 ounces	25	41
Beef steak, lean	3 ounces	24	44
Chicken, baked, no skin	3 ounces	24	60
Tuna in water	3 ounces	24	89
Salmon, broiled	3 ounces	23	50
Hamburger, regular	3 ounces	21	34
Shrimp	3 ounces	18	85
Yogurt, low-fat	1 cup	12	34
Whole milk	1 cup	9	23
Skim milk	1 cup	9	40
Milk, 2% fat	1 cup	8	26
Swiss cheese	1 ounce	8	30
Cheddar cheese	1 ounce	7	25
Egg	1 medium	6	32
Dried Beans and Nuts			
Soybeans, cooked	1 cup	20	38
Tofu	½ cup	10	43
Peanuts	¼ cup	9	17
Split peas, cooked	½ cup	8	28
Black or navy beans, cooked	½ cup	8	28
Peanut butter	2 tablespoons	8	17
Walnuts	¼ cup	8	14
Almonds	¼ cup	7	13
Lima beans, cooked	½ cup	5	24
Grains			
Noodles, cooked	1 cup	7	25
Corn	1 cup	5	29
Oatmeal, cooked	1 cup	5	15
Macaroni, cooked	1 cup	5	13
White rice, cooked	1 cup	4	11
Brown rice, cooked	1 cup	4	10
Whole-wheat bread	1 slice	2	15
White bread	1 slice	2	13

Fats in foods not only supply energy, but also fat-soluble nutrients. Fats carry essential fatty acids and the fat-soluble vitamins A, D, E, and K. So part of the reason that we need fats in our diets is to get a supply of the essential nutrients they carry. Fats are important to our taste buds in that fat increases the flavor of food. Fat in our body is used to cushion organs, help maintain a normal body temperature, and serve as a structural component of all cell membranes and nerves.

High fat intake is related to overweight and certain types of cancer. Diets high in saturated fats promote heart disease, especially in men. Primarily for these reasons, it is recommended that adults do not exceed 30 percent of total calories taken as fats. If you generally consume 1,600 calories, the maximum recommended number of grams of fat per day is 53 grams. If you consume 2,200 calories daily, it would be 73 grams, and at 2,800 calories, the maximum recommended intake of fat would be 93 grams. Diets containing 33 grams of fat or less per 1,000 calories provide 30 percent or less of total calories from fat. Nutrition information labels on food packages identify grams of fat in a serving of food and the percent of calories from fat. You can also refer to Table 2–4 for a listing of the fat content of common foods.

Cholesterol. Cholesterol is a close chemical relative of fat. It is a clear, oily liquid that is distributed in both the fatty and lean portions of many animal products. It is also produced by the human liver. Cholesterol is used by the body to form hormones and vitamin D, and is a component of all cell membranes. Beef, poultry, and seafood provide 30 to 80 mg of cholesterol per 3-ounce serving, whereas dairy products provide less than 30 mg per serving. Liver and eggs are the two richest sources of cholesterol in our diets. Cholesterol is not "fattening." It is not used by the body as a source of energy.

People are urged to consume less than 300 mg of cholesterol daily and most women do consume less than that amount. Actually, cholesterol intake is much more weakly associated with heart disease than is saturated fat intake. In addition, it is not clear whether high saturated fat and high cholesterol intake increase the risk of heart disease in most women.

Table 2-4 Food Sources of Fat

Food	Amount	Fat Content grams	Fat Content % of total calories
Fats and Oils			
Gravy	¼ cup	14	77
Mayonnaise	1 tablespoon	11	99
Heavy cream	1 tablespoon	6	93
Salad dressing	1 tablespoon	6	83
Oil	1 teaspoon	5	100
Butter	1 teaspoon	4	100
Margarine	1 teaspoon	4	100
Meats, Eggs			
Whopper	8.9 ounces	32	48
Big Mac	6.6 ounces	31	52
Quarter Pounder with cheese	6.8 ounces	29	50
Pork or beef with fat	3 ounces	18	62
Sausage	4 links	18	77
Hamburger, regular (20% fat)	3 ounces	17	62
Hot dog	1 (2 ounces)	17	83
Chicken, fried with skin	3 ounces	14	53
Salmon	3 ounces	11	46
Salami	2 ounces	11	68
Hamburger, lean (10% fat)	3 ounces	10	45
Steak (rib eye)	3 ounces	10	47
Steak (T-bone, lean)	3 ounces	9	44
Bacon	3 pieces	9	74
Bologna	1 ounce	8	80
Tuna in oil, drained	3 ounces	7	38
Egg	1	6	68
Steak (round, lean only)	3 ounces	5	29
Chicken, baked without skin	3 ounces	4	25
Venison	3 ounces	3	14
Hamburger, extra lean (4% fat)	3 ounces	2	23
Flounder, baked	3 ounces	1	13
Shrimp, boiled	3 ounces	1	7
Haddock	3 ounces	1	7

continued

Table 2–4 Food Sources of Fat, *continued*

Food	Amount	Fat Content grams	Fat Content % of total calories
Milk and Milk Products			
Cheddar cheese	1 ounce	9.5	74
Milk, whole	1 cup	8.5	49
American cheese	1 ounce	6.0	66
Cottage cheese, regular	½ cup	5.1	39
Milk, 2%	1 cup	5.0	32
Milk, 1%	1 cup	2.7	24
Cottage cheese, 1% fat	½ cup	1.2	13
Milk, skim	1 cup	0.4	4
Other			
French fries	20 fries	20.0	49
Walnuts	1 ounce	17.6	87
Peanuts	¼ cup	17.5	75
Sunflower seeds	¼ cup	17.0	77
Avocado	½	15.0	84
Almonds	1 ounce	15.0	80
Cashews	1 ounce	13.2	73
Potato chips	1 ounce (13 chips)	11.0	61
Chocolate chip cookies	4	11.0	54
Peanut butter	1 tablespoon	8.0	76
Taco chips	1 ounce (10 chips)	6.2	41
Mashed potatoes	½ cup	4.5	41
Olives	4 medium	1.5	90
Baked potato	1	0.2	1
Candy			
Mr. Goodbar	1.7 ounces	15.0	56
Peanut butter cups, 2 regular	1.6 ounces	15.0	54
Milk chocolate	1.6 ounces	14.0	53
Almond Joy	1.8 ounces	14.0	50
Twix	2.0 ounces	14.0	45
Baby Ruth	2.1 ounces	14.0	43
M and M's, peanut	1.7 ounces	13.0	47
Kit Kat	1.5 ounces	12.0	47
Snickers	2.1 ounces	13.0	42
Pay Day	1.9 ounces	12.0	43
Rolo, 10 candies	1.9 ounces	12.0	40
Butterfinger	2.1 ounces	12.0	39

continued

Table 2–4 Food Sources of Fat, *continued*

		Fat Content	
Food	Amount	grams	% of total calories
Sno-Caps	2.3 ounces	12.0	34
Nestle's Crunch	1.6 ounces	11.0	45
Milky Way	2.2 ounces	11.0	35
M and M's, plain	1.7 ounces	10.0	39
Whoppers	1.8 ounces	10.0	38
Three Musketeers	2.1 ounces	9.0	31
Raisinets	1.6 ounces	8.0	38
Milky Way II	2.2 ounces	5.5	26

Vitamins and Minerals

Humans require the thirteen vitamins and fifteen minerals listed in Table 2–5. If you see other substances labeled as vitamins or other minerals labeled as "essential," they are bogus. This rule applies, by the way, to lecithin, enzymes, co-enzymes, and other substances sold as essential for health but that the body produces.

Compared to the energy nutrients, vitamins and minerals are required in small amounts by the body. Vitamins facilitate the formation of energy in body tissues, and help protect the body from various diseases. Minerals serve as structural components of body tissues and are needed for the regulation of energy formation, nervous system function, and water balance.

Four of the vitamins are fat soluble (vitamins D, E, K, and A—or "Deka") while the other nine vitamins are water soluble. Because fat-soluble vitamins are stored in fat tissues, we generally have enough of these vitamins to last several months when dietary intake becomes low. With the exception of vitamin B_{12}, which can be stored in amounts that last for several years, the water-soluble vitamins are not stored in large amounts. Inadequate levels of intake of the water-soluble vitamins produce deficiency symptoms within a few weeks to a few months after dietary supply has stopped. If we fail to consume enough of each vitamin and essential mineral in our diets, specific deficiency diseases develop. On the other hand, if we consume excessive amounts of vitamins and minerals, overdose reactions occur.

Table 2–5 Vitamins and Minerals Required by Humans

Vitamins	Minerals
The B-complex vitamins:	Calcium
Thiamin (B_1)	Chloride
Riboflavin (B_2)	Chromium
Niacin (B_3)	Copper
B_6 (pyridoxine)	Fluoride
Folate (folacin, folic acid)	Iodine
B_{12} (cyanocobalamin)	Iron
Biotin	Magnesium
Pantothenic Acid (pantothenate)	Manganese
Vitamin C (ascorbic acid)	Molydbenum
Vitamin A (retinol)	Phosphorus
(provitamin is beta-carotene)	Potassium
Vitamin D (1,25 dihidroxy-colicalciferol)	Selenium
Vitamin E (tocopherol)	Sodium
Vitamin K (phylloquinone, menadione)	Zinc

The diverse functions of vitamins and minerals, as well as consequences of deficiency and overdose, major food sources, and other facts about vitamins and minerals are listed in Appendix B. In addition, Chapter 6 addresses vitamin and mineral supplement use in pregnancy.

Preserving the vitamin and mineral content of foods. Major losses of vitamins and minerals may occur during food storage and preparation. Overcooking, holding cooked foods on a warmer or steam table, and cooking foods in lots of water and tossing out the water that the foods are cooked in, all result in vitamin and mineral losses. (Overcooking vegetables should be a nutritional misdemeanor. In addition to causing vitamin and mineral losses, it tends to make people dislike vegetables!) Green beans and peas, if held hot for three hours before served, lose over half their content of thiamin, riboflavin, and vitamin C. Approximately one-third of the vitamin content of boiled vegetables is tossed out with the cooking water. Tips for preserving the vitamin and mineral content of foods are listed in Table 2–6.

Table 2–6 Food Storage and Preparation Methods that Preserve the Vitamin and Mineral Content of Foods

Storing Foods
- Store foods for the shortest amount of time possible.
- Choose fresh, freeze-dried, and frozen products over heavily processed and canned products.
- Store vegetables and fruits not needing refrigeration in a cool, dry, and clean place.
- Store leftover, perishable foods tightly wrapped in a refrigerator set just above 32°F.
- Avoid the freeze-thaw-freeze cycle. Foods defrosted, heated, and then refrozen show major losses in vitamin content.

Preparing Foods
- Don't overcook foods, especially vegetables. Cook most vegetables to the point where they are still a bit crunchy.
- Microwave, stir-fry, steam, or broil foods. Use just enough water to prevent scorching.
- Serve foods right after they have been prepared (or be the first one in the cafeteria line). Time food preparation so that the foods served are all ready at the same time.

Antioxidant nutrients. Beta carotene (a precursor of vitamin A), vitamins E and C, and selenium (an essential mineral) function as *antioxidants*. A variety of plant pigments and a number of enzymes produced by the body also function as antioxidants. These substances prevent or repair damage to cells caused by exposure to oxygen, ozone, smoke, and other oxidizing agents. Lack of sufficient levels of antioxidants in body tissues is related to premature aging, some types of cancer, bronchitis, emphysema, heart disease, cataracts, and pregnancy complications. People who consume five or more servings of fruits and vegetable each day tend to have better levels of intake of antioxidants than people who eat them less often.

Other important components of food. There is a wide variety of substances in food that are not required in our diets yet perform important functions in the body. We are just beginning to discover the health effects of compounds such as phenols in grape skins and wine, plant pigments (alpha-carotene, lycopene, and luetin, for example), and isoflavones in soy products. When regularly consumed, these substances appear to provide protection against a host of illnesses, including certain infectious diseases, heart disease, and some types of cancer. It is too soon to know with certainty the long-term health effects of these substances, or how much of them is best to consume. The recommendation that people eat five or more servings of fruits and vegetables daily is based, in part, on the benefits of these nonnutrient components of plant foods.

Recommended Levels of Nutrient Intake

The Recommended Dietary Allowances (RDAs) are the most widely used standard for identifying desired levels of essential nutrient intake (see Table 2–7).

Levels of intake set in the RDAs are sufficient to meet the needs of 98 percent of healthy people. A margin of safety is built into the RDAs, so intakes that are approximately 30 percent lower than the recommended level are likely sufficient. In general, consumption of essential nutrients and amounts up to twice the RDAs is considered safe.

A revised set of RDAs will be available by the year 2000. These new dietary intake standards will be called "Dietary Reference Intakes" and will include average nutrient requirements by age and gender, the recommended daily allowance, and intake levels above which the risk of overdose increases. Standards will be set for essential nutrients and other substances in foods known to influence health. (You can locate these new standards over the world-wide web at http://www2.nas.edu/fnb/215a.html.)

3. Poor Nutrition Can Result from Both Inadequate and Excessive Levels of Nutrient Intake

The main point of this principle is that you can become malnourished by consuming too little *or* too much of the nutrients. For each nutrient, there is a range of intake that is compatible with optimal functioning of the nutrient in the body. Up to a point, the body can adapt to low or high intakes of nutrients by using nutrient stores or by excreting excessive levels of nutrients through the urine or stools. Nutrient deficiency diseases or overdose symptoms

Table 2-7 Recommended Dietary Allowances (RDA), 1989[a]

Age (years)	Weight (kg)	Weight (lb)	Height (cm)	Height (inches)	Protein (g)	Vitamin A (RE)	Vitamin D (µg)	Vitamin E (mg)	Vitamin K (µg)	Vitamin C (mg)	Thiamin (mg)	Riboflavin (mg)	Niacin (mg equiv.)	Vitamin B6 (mg)	Folate (µg)	Vitamin B12 (µg)	Calcium (mg)	Phosphorus (mg)	Magnesium (mg)	Iron (mg)	Zinc (mg)	Iodine (µg)	Selenium (µg)
Infants
0.0–0.5	6	13	60	24	13	375	7.5	3	5	30	0.3	0.4	5	0.3	25	0.3	400	300	40	6	5	40	10
0.5–1.0	9	20	71	28	14	375	10	4	10	35	0.4	0.5	6	0.6	35	0.5	600	500	60	10	5	50	15
Children
1–3	13	29	90	35	16	400	10	6	15	40	0.7	0.8	9	1.0	50	0.7	800	800	80	10	10	70	20
4–6	20	44	112	44	24	500	10	7	20	45	0.9	1.1	12	1.1	75	1.0	800	800	120	10	10	90	20
7–10	28	62	132	52	28	700	10	7	30	45	1.0	1.2	13	1.4	100	1.4	800	800	170	10	10	120	30
Males
11–14	45	99	157	62	45	1000	10	10	45	50	1.3	1.5	17	1.7	150	2.0	1200	1200	270	12	15	150	40
15–18	66	145	176	69	59	1000	10	10	65	60	1.5	1.8	20	2.0	200	2.0	1200	1200	400	12	15	150	50
19–24	72	160	177	70	58	1000	10	10	70	60	1.5	1.7	19	2.0	200	2.0	1200	1200	350	10	15	150	70
25–50	79	174	176	70	63	1000	5	10	80	60	1.5	1.7	19	2.0	200	2.0	800	800	350	10	15	150	70
51+	77	170	173	68	63	1000	5	10	80	60	1.2	1.4	15	2.0	200	2.0	800	800	350	10	15	150	70

continued

Table 2-7 Recommended Dietary Allowances (RDA), 1989[a], *continued*

Age (years)	Weight (kg)	Weight (lb)	Height (cm)	Height (inches)	Protein (g)	Vitamin A (RE)	Vitamin D (µg)	Vitamin E (mg)	Vitamin K (µg)	Vitamin C (mg)	Thiamin (mg)	Riboflavin (mg)	Niacin (mg equiv.)	Vitamin B$_6$ (mg)	Folate (µg)	Vitamin B$_{12}$ (µg)	Calcium (mg)	Phosphorus (mg)	Magnesium (mg)	Iron (mg)	Zinc (mg)	Iodine (µg)	Selenium (µg)
Females																							
11–14	46	101	157	62	46	800	10	8	45	50	1.1	1.3	15	1.4	150	2.0	1200	1200	280	15	12	150	45
15–18	55	120	163	64	44	800	10	8	55	60	1.1	1.3	15	1.5	180	2.0	1200	1200	300	15	12	150	50
19–24	58	128	164	65	46	800	10	8	60	60	1.1	1.3	15	1.6	180	2.0	1200	1200	280	15	12	150	55
25–50	63	138	163	64	50	800	5	8	65	60	1.1	1.3	15	1.6	180	2.0	800	800	280	15	12	150	55
51+	65	143	160	63	50	800	5	8	65	60	1.0	1.2	13	1.6	180	2.0	800	800	280	10	12	150	55
Pregnant					60	800	10	10	65	70	1.5	1.6	17	2.2	400	2.2	1200	1200	320	30	15	175	65
Lactating																							
1st 6 months					65	1300	10	12	65	95	1.6	1.8	20	2.1	280	2.6	1200	1200	355	15	19	200	75
2nd 6 months					62	1200	10	11	65	90	1.6	1.7	20	2.1	260	2.6	1200	1200	340	15	16	200	75

[a]The allowances are intended to provide for individual variations among most normal, healthy people in the United States under usual environmental stresses. Diets should be based on a variety of common foods in order to provide other nutrients for which human requirements have been less well defined.

Source: Reprinted with permission from *Recommended Dietary Allowances,* 10th ed. Copyright 1989 by the National Academy of Sciences. Courtesy of the National Academy Press, Washington, D.C.

result when we exceed the body's capacity to adjust for low or high levels of intake. If we consume too little vitamin C, for example, the body calls upon its limited store of vitamin C and when this runs out, signs of a deficiency begin to develop. Deficiency symptoms may start within as little as a month without vitamin C intake. The first sign of a deficiency is usually delayed wound healing. If allowed to progress, the vitamin C deficiency leads to gums that bleed easily, pain and bruising upon being touched, and abnormal bone growth. Excessive intake of vitamin C (a gram or more daily) produces diarrhea and may contribute to the development of kidney stones. Nearly all cases of vitamin or mineral overdose result from the excessive use of supplements.

4. Malnutrition Can Be Caused by Poor Diets or Diseased States

People can become malnourished due to inadequate or excessive levels of nutrient intake or because body functions are impaired due to an inherited condition, surgery, disease, or certain medications. Bleeding ulcers, for example, are a common cause of iron deficiency in the elderly. People who have a condition that causes the storage of too much iron suffer from iron overdose. Impairments in bodily functions in people with cancer and HIV/AIDS frequently lead to malnutrition.

5. Some Groups of People Are at Higher Risk of Becoming Malnourished Than Others

The risk of malnutrition is not shared equally among all people. Individuals with a high need for nutrients due to pregnancy, breastfeeding, growth, illness, or recovery from illness or surgery will develop malnutrition faster in times of food shortage than will healthy people. In cases of widespread famine, such as that induced by natural disasters or war, the health of nutritionally vulnerable groups is compromised soonest and most. The younger the person at the time of a food shortage, and the longer the shortage of food exists, the more lasting are the ill effects on health and mental development.

6. Poor Nutrition Can Influence the Development of Certain Chronic Diseases

Vitamin and mineral deficiency and overdose diseases are not the only health problems related to poor nutrition. Faulty diets play important roles in the development of heart disease, hypertension, diabetes, cancer, osteoporosis, dental disease, poor pregnancy outcomes, and other disorders. In general, diets high in animal fat and low in vegetables and fruits are related to the development of these chronic diseases.

7. Adequacy and Balance Are Key Characteristics of Healthy Diets

Healthy diets contain many different foods that together provide calories and nutrients in amounts that promote health. Variety is a cornerstone of an adequate and balanced diet because no one food (except breast milk for young infants) provides all the nutrients we need. Most foods don't even come close to doing that.

Healthy diets are built around foods, not supplements, because there are many healthful substances in basic foods that are not available in supplements. If there is a choice between foods and supplements, you should choose foods first.

Building Healthy Diets

Take a moment to relax, close your eyes for a second, and take a deep breath. Now, give your full attention to these foods:

- A plump, golden peach. It's so ripe that juices spurt from it and drip down your chin when you take a bite.
- A Thanksgiving turkey. It's still in the oven roasting, and the wonderful smell fills the whole kitchen.
- A steaming loaf of golden-brown homemade bread that has just been set out to cool.
- A perfectly ripe, just-picked tomato that melts in your mouth.

If your mouth is watering and you are ready to go out and buy some ripe peaches, you have found the balance between good taste and good for you.

Eating a healthy diet has to mean eating food you enjoy. If it doesn't, or if it's too much of a struggle, a diet won't last. Healthy diets are those people can live with and enjoy for a lifetime. The trick to getting one going that will last is planning and choosing foods you like that are nutritious.

Proper diets are made up of the collection of foods we eat over the course of a day or several days. It's the sum of the contributions made by individual foods that produces a diet that is either healthy or not. This means that there are no single foods (other than spoiled meat or poison mushrooms) that are "bad" for you or others that are "good." As Hippocrates pointed out, diets are relatively good or bad.

Dietary Guidelines for Americans

To help consumers decide what constitutes a healthy diet, "Dietary Guidelines for Americans" have been developed and are periodically updated. You can obtain a free, forty-three-page brochure on these guidelines by writing to the address given at the end of the book, or you can obtain a copy through the Internet. The Dietary Guidelines for Americans provide the rationale for a healthy diet and urge Americans to:

- Eat a variety of foods
- Balance the foods eaten with physical activity—maintain or improve weight
- Choose a diet with plenty of grain products, vegetables, and fruits
- Choose a diet low in fat, saturated fat, and cholesterol
- Choose a diet moderate in sugars
- Choose a diet moderate in salt and sodium
- Drink alcoholic beverages in moderation, if at all

The Food Guide Pyramid (The Four Basic Food Groups)

How do you select the combination of foods that add up to a healthy diet? One straightforward way is to build diets around the recommended number of servings from the basic food groups and the Food Guide Pyramid (see Figure 2–1).

This guide encourages people to eat from the base of the pyramid up, or to eat lower on the food chain. The Food Guide Pyramid recommends a range of servings per day from each of the basic food groups. To use this guide, however, you need to know

Figure 2–1 Food Guide Pyramid

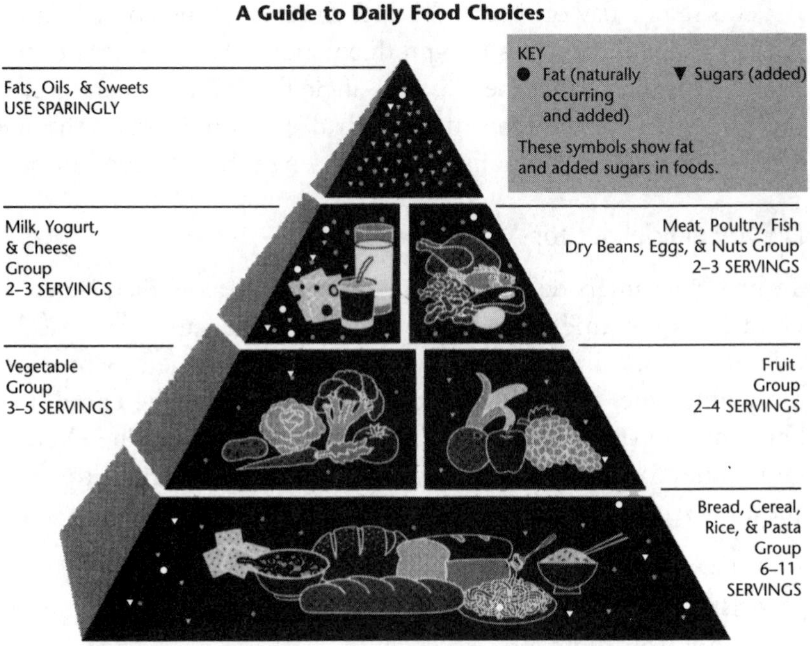

A Guide to Daily Food Choices

KEY
● Fat (naturally occurring and added) ▼ Sugars (added)

These symbols show fat and added sugars in foods.

Fats, Oils, & Sweets
USE SPARINGLY

Milk, Yogurt, & Cheese Group
2–3 SERVINGS

Meat, Poultry, Fish Dry Beans, Eggs, & Nuts Group
2–3 SERVINGS

Vegetable Group
3–5 SERVINGS

Fruit Group
2–4 SERVINGS

Bread, Cereal, Rice, & Pasta Group
6–11 SERVINGS

Source: U.S. Department of Agriculture/U.S. Department of Health and Human Services

what a standard serving size is. Table 2–8 lists standard serving sizes referred to in the Food Guide Pyramid.

The Food Guide Pyramid can be used for very practical applications such as planning grocery lists and meals, and for ordering off a restaurant menu. There are many types of foods included in each food group. You can pick your favorites from the choices listed in Table 2–9.

Combination dishes such as chili, moussaka, chicken stew, ratatouille, and soup are not listed in this table. However, basic foods can be combined in many ways to make interesting and tasty dishes that fit nicely into healthy diets.

A healthy diet doesn't have to omit all sweets and high-calorie snacks, but it does mean limiting them to reasonable amounts. Diets

Table 2–8 What Counts as One Serving?

Food Group	Serving Size
A. Bread, Cereal, Rice, and Pasta	
Bread	1 slice
Rice, cooked	½ cup
Pasta	½ cup
Hot cereal	½ cup
Grits	½ cup
Cold cereal	1 cup
Granola	¼ cup
Tortilla	1
Chapati	1
Bagel	½
English muffin	½
Crackers	3 to 4 small
Muffin	½ (1 ounce)
Waffle	1 small
Pancake	1 small
Roll	1 small
B. Vegetables	
Raw or cooked	½ cup
Leafy	1 cup
Vegetable juice	¾ cup
C. Fruits	
Fruit, fresh	1
Cantaloupe	⅛ whole
Fruit, canned	½ cup
Applesauce	½ cup
Dried fruit	¼ cup
Berries, fresh	1 cup
Fruit juice	¾ cup
D. Milk	
Milk	1 cup
Fortified soy milk	1 cup
Yogurt	1 cup
Cottage cheese	½ cup
Cheese	1½ ounces

continued

Table 2–8 What Counts as One Serving? *continued*

Food Group	Serving Size
E. Meat, Poultry, Fish, Dry Beans, Eggs, and Nuts	
Meat, poultry, fish	3 ounces
Dried beans, cooked	½ cup
Tofu	½ cup
Seeds	½ cup
Eggs	2
Peanut butter	4 tablespoons
F. Miscellaneous, Fats, Oils, Sweets	
Butter	2 teaspoons
Margarine	2 teaspoons
Salad dressing	2 tablespoons
Sweets	1 ounce
Alcoholic beverage	1

that are based on the food groups usually have room for a serving or two a day of foods you eat mostly for fun. Because of their high caloric needs, very physically active people, pregnant and breastfeeding women, and children may need the calories provided by snacks and desserts.

Vegetarian Diets

If vegetarians eat plants, what do humanitarians eat?

There are many variations of vegetarian diets. Some people who don't eat red meat, or eat only fish and plant foods consider themselves to be vegetarians. In its truest sense, a vegetarian diet includes only plant foods.

There are a number of benefits to eating low on the food chain. Vegetarians tend to have a lower risk of heart disease, cancer, obesity, and Type II (noninsulin-dependent) diabetes than meat eaters. The fact that many vegetarians do not smoke or drink alcohol excessively, and engage in regular physical activity, likely contributes to their maintenance of good health.

Vegetarian diets generally contain less protein than the average American diet, but nonetheless an adequate amount. (In other

Table 2–9 Basic Food Choices by Food Group

A. Bread, Cereal, Rice, Pastas

bagel	crackers	pancakes	rice cakes
biscuits	granola	polenta	rolls
bread (any type)	grits	pretzels	tortillas
cold cereals	hot cereals	popcorn	waffles
corn bread	muffins	rice	wild rice

B. Vegetables

asparagus	cauliflower	leeks	rutabagas
bean sprouts	coleslaw	lettuce (any type)	spinach
beets	collard greens	lima beans	squash
black-eyed peas	corn	mushrooms	sweet potatoes
broccoli	cucumber	okra	tomato
brussels sprouts	eggplant	onions	tomato juice
cabbage	green beans	peppers (any type)	turnips
carrots	green peas	potatoes	vegetable juice

C. Fruits

apples	cantaloupe	honeydew melon	pineapple
apple juice	cherries	kiwi fruit	pineapple juice
applesauce	cranberry juice	mango	plums
apricots	fruit cocktail	orange	raspberries
avocado	grapefruit	papaya	strawberries
banana	grapefruit juice	peach	watermelon
blueberries	grapes	pear	

D. Meat, Poultry, Fish, Dry Beans, Eggs, and Nuts

1. Animal Products

beef (lean)	egg substitute	lobster	turkey
chicken	fish (any type)	pork	veal
crab	ham	scallops	
eggs	lamb	shrimp	

2. Plant Products

dried beans	nuts (any type)	soy milk (fortified)	tofu
hummus	peanut butter	split pea	
lentils	seeds (any type)	tempeh	

E. Milk, Yogurt, and Cheese

cheese (any type)	frozen yogurt	milk
cottage cheese	ice milk	yogurt

F. Fats, Oils, Sweets, and Alcohol

beer	candy	cookies	salad dressing
butter	chocolate	margarine	wine

words, vegetarians tend to overconsume protein less than most other Americans.) The adequate but relatively low protein intake of vegetarians has the side benefit of reducing the requirement for calcium. High-protein diets lead to losses of calcium through the urine.

Vegetarian diet precautions. There is such a thing as unhealthful vegetarian diets. Vegetarian diets can include too many high-calorie foods such as French fries, candy, desserts, and pastries. If limited in variety, vegetarian diets can produce deficiencies of many nutrients, but in particular, iron, zinc, calcium, vitamin B_{12}, and vitamin D. Vegetarians who do not consume fortified soy milk may need to take a vitamin supplement in order to get sufficient levels of vitamin B_{12} and vitamin D. Vitamin B_{12} is only found in animal products and fortified foods. Fermented foods such as spirulina, seaweed, and tempeh have been touted as good sources of vitamin B_{12}. However, as much as 94 percent of the form of vitamin B_{12} found in these foods is inactive. Vitamin D is found only in a few foods, of which the leading source is vitamin D–fortified cows' milk. (Other dairy products such as yogurt and cheese are not fortified with vitamin D.) This vitamin is produced by the body from cholesterol when the skin is exposed to sunlight. Vegetarians who do not consume vitamin D–fortified milk, fortified soy milk, or fortified cereals, or who do not expose their skin to regular sunshine, are at risk of poor bone formation and maintenance due to vitamin D deficiency. Enough sun exposure for maintaining vitamin D production in the skin is about fifteen to thirty minutes on the arms, hands, and legs three to four times a week. Glass and sunscreen block the sun's ultraviolet rays and the skin's manufacture of vitamin D. One other note: the intensity of the sun's rays in northern climates in the winter is insufficient for production of vitamin D. You have to take a tropical vacation each winter to get your vitamin D. . . .

Well-planned vegetarian diets are adequate for pregnant and breast-feeding women and for infants after the age of four to six months. Before that time, infants should be exclusively breast-fed or given iron-fortified infant formula. Care should also be taken in the diet to include sufficient calories and vitamins B_{12} and D, and calcium, iron, and zinc.

Recipes for Quick Nutritious Meals

Diets based on the food groups can take the form of delicious and nutritious beverages, appetizers, entrees, side dishes, and desserts. We have placed a mini-cookbook of tested recipes in Appendix A of this book to give you examples of nutritious dishes that are easily prepared. Recipes for both vegetarians and meat eaters are included. Most recipes take about thirty minutes to prepare, and they are nearly all low in fat and come with an analysis of caloric and nutrient content.

Diagnosing the Truthfulness of Nutrition Information

Deciding whether something you read or hear about dietary supplements or nutritional remedies can be difficult. The marketplace is replete with products that promise to raise children's IQ, build muscle, melt fat, cure infection, and restore lost energy. Unlike drugs, products sold as foods or dietary supplements do not have to be tested for safety or effectiveness before they are offered to the public. Some products, such as certain herbs and high doses of vitamins and minerals, are not safe for everyone, however. Although promoters of nutritional products are not supposed to make untrue claims, it happens all the time. Untested promises for dietary supplements, weight-loss aids, and herbal remedies are commonly made by salespeople. Purported benefits of nutritional products are touted in pamphlets, advertisements, infomercials, and on TV and radio talk shows. There is little enforcement of existing regulations that prohibit bogus claims and the mild penalties applied for wrongdoing make the risk of false statements largely worth it. The potential for lawsuits for personal injury appears to represent the strongest disincentive for offering unsafe or ineffective products. Because of the lack of enforcement of protective regulations, consumers are truly on their own to decide if what they hear or read about nutritional remedies or other products is true.

How, then, do you decide if something you read or hear about nutrition is true, or, at a minimum, safe to try? Here are some suggestions for sorting out nutrition facts from fiction.

Be suspicious of the money motive. Products heavily advertised in Sunday newspaper supplements, in tabloids, and in-flight magazines, or on radio or television that offer "new," "revolutionary," or "breakthrough" nutritional products are highly suspect. Such heavy investments in advertising spell *profit motive*. If the product worked, it wouldn't have to be oversold in such detail in advertisements. Products that offer a money-back guarantee are also suspect. Only the rare consumer returns a product even if it doesn't really work for anyone. There is no need to offer your money back if a product does what it claims to do.

Testimonials are a strong clue that a nutritional product is bogus. Testimonials are worthless, regardless of what degrees or how many movies the speaker has to his or her credit. Nutritional products are a business and people get paid to help promote them. The commonly used before-and-after photographs of people using particular weight-loss products have employed different subjects in the before and the after photographs. Well-respected scientists in areas other than nutrition have been given sizable research grants as payment for support of specific, unproven nutritional products.

Only objective research can determine whether a product does what is claimed. Because many consumers are aware of this, advertisements will often announce that the product has been extensively tested and has been shown by research to work. If that is the case, write to the manufacturer and ask for a copy of the published studies. If the appropriate studies have been done, the papers could be sent. Chances are excellent, however, that you will not hear back from the manufacturers who touted the scientific studies.

There are several reasons why so many untested nutritional products are available. Studies needed to test the effectiveness and safety of products are expensive. Even if they are undertaken and a product found to be beneficial, most of the ingredients of nutritional products could not be patented. Ingredients such as vitamins, minerals, herbs, enzymes, amino acids, and algae are not unique discoveries and can be used in products by any manufacturer.

Formulations of nutritional ingredients can be patented, however.

Overall, the current situation provides little incentive for manufacturers of nutritional products to invest in research. The lack of effectiveness of most of the products offered to the public insures that there will be a continuing market for new, revolutionary formulas in the future. After all, if these remedies worked, there would be no need for additional products.

Sometimes people who represent nutritional remedies are sincere and convinced of the benefits of the products they sell despite the lack of objective proof. The problem here is that you cannot know whether the product is a bad or a good investment. You have to treat all such claims as suspect until you are shown that they are not. The standard of proof has to be the results of scientific studies. Otherwise, you cannot predict the safety or effectiveness of nutritional products. Insisting on proof that a nutritional product is safe and actually does what it is claimed to do is really not asking that much.

Reliable Sources of Nutrition Information

Not all the nutrition information you read in newspapers, books, or magazines, or hear on radio or TV, is nonsense. Many periodicals and broadcasting companies are cautious about the accuracy of information presented. This caution is exercised by investigating the reliability of the sources of nutrition information, by covering more than one side of controversial topics, and by confirming conclusions with nutrition experts before the information is presented. Some print and broadcasting companies have policies that reject advertisements that make false or deceptive nutrition claims.

Reliable nutrition information can be found in:

- Government health publications
- Information produced by scientifically recognized professional organizations such as the American Dietetic Association, the American Institute of Nutrition, and the American Medical Association; professional and voluntary associations such as the American Heart Association or the March of Dimes also provide reliable nutrition information
- Articles in scientific journals that primarily publish research studies

- College nutrition textbooks
- Books written by scientifically credible experts in nutrition

Other reliable sources of nutrition information exist, but it is impossible to give them blank approval because the credibility of the data presented varies too much. For example, popular nutrition books written by people with impressive backgrounds in another field may contain hogwash, or they may be accurate. You can't tell by the credentials of the author alone. Nor can you always trust information relayed in "educational" publications produced by the food and dietary supplement industry. Infant formula companies; organizations representing the meat, wheat, potato, and dairy industries; manufacturers of vitamins and mineral supplements; and a host of other organizations publish nutrition information to promote their products. Some of these publications can be found in the waiting rooms of health care providers. Sometimes the nutrition information conveyed is accurate, but often it is slanted in favor of the company's products. Advertisements may be included along with the articles on nutrition, and the topics selected for coverage commonly relate only to the type of food, vitamins, or other products sold by the sponsoring company.

Much of the information in this section relates to claims about nutrition and health that lie outside of what is known to be true. The truth, however, has a lot going for it—it's what you can count on.

This is the end of your "crash course" on nutrition and background information for the upcoming recommendations. If you would like to learn more about nutrition, enroll in a class at a nearby college, check out a nutrition textbook from the library, or take a self-study course. The subject is more complex than one might think and we are learning more about it every day. Take advantage of the knowledge.

⁓ 3 ⁓

Nutrition and Fertility

To bring on the menses, recover the flesh by giving a woman puddings, roast meats, a good wine, fresh air, and sun.

—Advice on the treatment of infertility, 1847

Nutrition has long been suspected of playing a role in fertility, but it has only been during the last twenty years that specific relationships have been scientifically documented. It is now clear that dietary habits, weight status, and supplement use can directly affect a woman's chances of conceiving. The nutritional remedies for infertility suggested here are inexpensive and safe, and although they will not correct all cases of infertility, they represent underused potential solutions.

It is easy to become amazed by the complexity of the biological processes involved in fertility. For conception to occur, hundreds of interdependent biological processes must function in harmony. Defects in any one process can prevent or delay conception. When you consider all that could go awry, it is truly remarkable that conception ever occurs.

If pregnancy does not occur within twelve months of unprotected intercourse, a diagnosis of infertility is usually made. Using this standard definition, one in six couples in the United States are infertile. A history of conception or pregnancy does not guarantee that an individual or couple is fertile. About half of all cases of infertility occur after one or more pregnancies. Infertility may not be forever. Conception eventually occurs without medical intervention in approximately half of all couples who fail to conceive within twelve months of attempting pregnancy.

The diagnosis and treatment of infertility is frequently a challenge because information about its causes is incomplete. Defects in sperm production, tubal obstruction, a history of pelvic inflammatory disease, anabolic steroid abuse, and hormone abnormalities are all related to infertility. Women over the age of thirty-five are at higher risk for infertility and delayed conception than are younger women. Infertility and delayed conception in women are also related to a number of nutritional factors:

- underweight
- obesity
- famine/dieting
- high caffeine consumption
- alcohol use
- vitamin and mineral supplement use
- eating disorders
- vegetarian diets

These factors likely account for a portion of cases of infertility of unknown cause and those linked to hormonal abnormalities. Unfortunately, nutritional links to infertility are often not assessed clinically. They should be, however, because cases of nutrition-related infertility can be corrected if appropriate changes in body weight or diet are made. "Low-tech" ways of correcting infertility through modifications in nutritional status are addressed below.

Body Weight and Fertility

Estrogen is a hormone that plays a major role in reproduction. It is produced in two places in the body: the ovaries and the fat stores. Low or high levels of body fat, and a tendency to store fat centrally (around the waistline) all change estrogen production. These modifications in estrogen production can lead to infertility or a delay in conception due to a loss of menstrual periods or a lack of ovulation (egg release). The amount and location of body fat may also alter the production of other reproductive hormones in ways that decrease fertility.

A number of studies have demonstrated a normalization of reproductive hormone levels and a correction of infertility after body fat
content is brought closer to the normal range. Weight loss as modest
as 14 pounds among obese, infertile women through a reduction in
caloric intake and an increase in physical activity has been shown to
correct infertility in a majority of women studied. Weight loss generally reduces central body fat stores and lessens the risk of infertility and delayed conception related to a waistline pattern of fat storage.
Although ovulation and normal hormonal levels can sometimes
medically be induced in underweight and obese women, infant outcomes tend to be better if ovulation is achieved spontaneously.

What Is Too Much or Too Little Body Fat?

As a general rule, individuals who have less than 20 percent or
greater than 30 percent of their total weight as fat are too lean or
too fat, respectively. By weight for height these levels are less than
90 percent or over 130 percent of average weight for height. Table
3–1 shows average weights for height and weights that correspond
to underweight or obesity. The risk of infertility or delayed conception increases as the extent of underweight or obesity increases.
However, weights for height up to 130 percent of standard do not
appear to be related to infertility.

Body weight, while often a reliable measure, isn't always a good
indicator of how lean or fat a person is. Individuals who exercise a
lot may weigh in the normal or overweight range but actually be
too lean because of a low percentage of body fat. On the other
hand, people who are sedentary may be normal weight but have too
much body fat. It is for these individuals that weight standards may
not be a good indicator of body fatness. As a rough guide, if you can
pinch over an inch or more of fat lying under the skin around your
waist or back of your upper arm, you probably have excessive body
fat. Underfat women will pinch less than half an inch at these sites.

Waist circumference is considered a good measure of central
body fat stores. A waist circumference of 39 inches or more represents an excessive level of central body fat in most women, regardless of height.

Table 3-1 Weight for Height Standards for Women*

Height (without shoes)	Average weight (without clothes)	Underweight (<90% of average)	Obese (>130% of average)
4' 9"	100	90	130
4' 10"	103	93	134
4' 11"	106	95	138
5' 0"	109	98	142
5' 1"	112	101	146
5' 2"	116	104	151
5' 3"	120	108	156
5' 4"	124	112	161
5' 5"	128	115	166
5' 6"	132	119	172
5' 7"	136	122	177
5' 8"	140	126	182
5' 9"	144	130	187
5'10"	148	133	192
5'11"	152	137	198
6'0"	156	140	203
6' 1"	160	144	208
6' 2"	165	149	215

* Adopted from the 1959 Metropolitan Life Insurance tables for women 25 years of age and older.

Famine, Dieting, and Fertility

It has been known for decades that one of the first effects of famine on populations is reduced fertility. When food becomes available again, normal rates of fertility return within the population. This scenario makes sense in that undernourished women are ill prepared to sustain a growing fetus.

Part of the reason infertility follows famine is a loss of body fat reserves. But an abrupt decline in caloric intake may also impair fertility in women not experiencing famine. Low caloric intake results in absent or irregular ovulation that may prevent or delay conception. When infertility or delayed conception is related to low calorie diets, normal fertility returns after intake becomes adequate.

Caffeine Consumption and Fertility

Intakes of over 300 mg caffeine per day, the equivalent of over two cups of brewed coffee, appear to be weakly related to infertility and delayed conception. Coffee intake of two or fewer cups per day appear to be unrelated to fertility. The relationship between caffeine intake and fertility is termed "weak" because some studies show no relationship while other results demonstrate a small effect. One study concluded that high caffeine intake may benefit fertility. It is not clear whether caffeine, something else in coffee, or character- istics of coffee drinkers are responsible for the relationship.

Should you cut back or stop drinking coffee if fertility or delayed conception is a concern? The reasonable response for now is "yes," even though it may or may not help. Regular coffee drinkers should be prepared for "caffeine withdrawal" headaches if they abruptly cut down on coffee. Should you reduce intake of all sources of caffeine or just coffee? The answer to this question depends on whether you are consuming over 300 mg caffeine daily from other sources of caffeine.

Certain teas have a good deal of caffeine and may elevate total caffeine intake to beyond 300 mg daily. Herbal teas generally don't contain caffeine. Package labels often include information on the caffeine content of the tea. In addition, chocolate and many soft drinks contain caffeine. See Table 3–2.

Alcohol and Fertility

Heavy drinking appears to be related to infertility, but the con- sumption of one or two drinks of alcohol-containing beverages daily does not. Since alcohol consumption within the first two months after conception may harm the fetus, women are advised to abstain from drinking if they might conceive.

Vitamin and Mineral Supplement Use and Fertility

There is limited information that suggests a multivitamin and min- eral supplement may improve fertility. A European study involving

Table 3–2 Caffeine Content of Beverages

	Caffeine (mg)
Coffee, 1 cup	
drip	137–153
percolated	97–125
instant	61–70
decaffeinated	0–4
Tea, 1 cup	
imported	40–176
U.S. brands	32–144
instant, iced tea	40–80
Soft drinks, 12 ounces	
Mountain Dew	54
Diet Cola	46
Dr. Pepper	40
Coca-Cola	38
Pepsi-Cola	38
Diet Pepsi	37
Ginger ale	0
7-Up	0
Cocoa or chocolate milk, 1 cup	10–17

thousands of women attempting pregnancy found that those who took a multivitamin and mineral supplement conceived sooner than other women. It is possible that the supplements improved women's nutritional status and reproductive system function. There is some evidence that iron deficiency impairs fertility; therefore, the vitamin and mineral supplement may have corrected that problem.

It is not recommended that women or men take a multivitamin and mineral supplement or any other type of supplement to aid conception. However, nutrient amounts in supplements labeled as "100 percent of the daily value" are safe for the vast majority of people. Use of high amounts of vitamins or minerals in supplements (or dose levels beyond 100 percent) is not recommended, primarily because of the potential for adverse effects on the fetus very early in pregnancy. The exception to this recommendation is folic acid, which may be needed in high amounts by women who have had a baby with a neural tube defect such as spina bifida. (See Chapter 6 for additional information on this topic.)

Eating Disorders and Fertility

Women with anorexia nervosa, bulimia, or a combination of these problems are less likely to conceive and maintain a pregnancy than are women who do not have an eating disorder. Lowered fertility results from low levels of body fat in some women and possibly from alterations in reproductive hormones due to other causes. Restoration of weight and an end to binge-purge cycles improves fertility. It is especially important that normal eating habits and weight gain are maintained throughout pregnancy.

Vegetarian Diets and Fertility

Women who consume plants only tend to take longer to conceive than meat eaters. The reason appears to be longer menstrual cycles and less frequent ovulation in some vegans. It is suspected that a high intake of plant estrogens and fiber or a low fat intake may be responsible for hormonal changes that increase cycle length. Vegans do not tend to be infertile. Rather, vegans may take longer than average to conceive because ovulation is less frequent when menstrual cycles are further apart.

Nutrition and Male Fertility

About half of all cases of infertility are male related, yet far less is known about nutritional relationships to fertility in men than in women. It is known that low or high levels of body fat, famine, and weight loss affect sperm production in men, and that excessive alcohol consumption and anabolic steroid use reduces male fertility. Other threats to male fertility include DDT, PCB, and heavy metal (lead, cadmium, manganese) exposure from the environment. The cycle of sperm development imposes a three-month delay in the appearance of fertility impairments due to these exposures. Recovery from short-term exposures also takes about three months.

Subfertility

Sometimes women have normal fertility or experience conception as expected, but for some reason their pregnancies are not maintained. When three or more conceptions end early due to resorption of an embryo (or the absorption of an embryo into the uterine wall) or miscarriage, "subfertility" is said to exist. Actually, resorption of an embryo and miscarriage are relatively common events. It is estimated that 50 to 60 percent of all conceptions are lost early in pregnancy. Between 22 and 44 percent of losses occur before the diagnosis of pregnancy is made; 6 to 13 percent take place between pregnancy diagnosis and the twenty-eighth week of pregnancy. Although women who have experienced an early loss may not take comfort in these statistics, resorptions and miscarriages are, unfortunately, common events.

Early pregnancy losses can be due to congenital malformations, reproductive tract infections, and severe trauma. They are more likely to occur in women who do not experience nausea or nausea and vomiting early in pregnancy, who are over the age of thirty-five, or who work in physically demanding jobs. Consumption of more than two cups of coffee a day or two drinks of alcohol-containing beverages per week in the first two months of pregnancy have been associated with miscarriage. It is suspected that underweight and weight loss early in pregnancy may be related to miscarriage in some women.

☙ 4 ☙

Becoming Nutritionally Prepared for the First Two Months of Pregnancy

Everyone is kneaded out of the same dough, but not baked in the same oven.

—Yiddish proverb

U ntil recently, it was widely believed that the most important time for paying attention to nutrition was in the last half of pregnancy when the fetus was gaining most of its birth weight. It was assumed that the importance of nutrition in pregnancy grew along with the fetus. The emphasis on nutrition later in pregnancy made sense because that is what had been studied and its importance was clear. It was also practical, since most women did not receive prenatal care until well into pregnancy. This situation is changing as results of new studies become available and as interest in preconceptional and early pregnancy care grows among obstetric providers and women. New information is demonstrating that nutrition during the first few months of pregnancy is of more importance than had been previously imagined. The information represents an exciting advance because, if women know about it, they can apply much of the new information before they begin prenatal care.

Preconception and early pregnancy nutrition are attracting a high level of attention because of research results showing the effects of nutrition on fetal tissue and organ formation, and on health long after delivery. Since most fetal tissues and organs develop within the first two months of pregnancy, waiting until pregnancy is confirmed to make changes in nutritional practices may mean opportunities are missed. To take full advantage of the benefits of good nutrition, it is best to practice optimal nutrition before conception. That way, when conception occurs, you will be nutritionally set for the critically important first months of pregnancy.

This chapter takes you on a brief tour of early fetal development and growth and describes how a woman's body changes to accommodate pregnancy. Preconception and early pregnancy nutritional practices that support optimal fetal development and growth are described and specific recommendations given.

The First Two Months of Pregnancy

Each of us began life as a single cell. That phase of life lasted a very short time, however. Shortly after conception, the single fertilized cell burst into action by dividing and creating new cells. By the time of birth, one cell had multiplied into trillions of cells. Not each cell became an exact replica of the other. Although each cell contains the same genetic material, groups of cells developed specialized functions along the way. This specialization allowed cells to form specific tissues and organs that would perform particular functions. Our brains are able to remember and to reason, and our bodies can digest food, eliminate waste, combat infection, renew bone, and perform thousands of other functions because groups of cells develop differently from other groups.

Not all tissues and organs were formed by groups of specialized cells at the same time. There was a preprogrammed time for development for every tissue and organ in our bodies. Our spinal cords, which developed into our brains, were formed within twenty-three days after conception. By thirty days after conception, in each of us a cluster of cells had formed a heart that beat weakly. Arms, legs, fingers, and toes had also taken shape by then. Within two more weeks, groups of cells had formed basic components of the liver, pancreas, stomach, ears, eyes, and lungs. All these miraculous accomplishments occurred before the cluster of cells, referred to as the embryo, weighed 5 grams, or the weight of a nickel! Each tissue and organ had to develop on schedule because there was no second chance. Development is on a very strict timetable.

In order for tissues and organs to form and function normally, all building materials must be present at the time tissues and organs are programmed to develop. If sufficient oxygen, water, glucose, vitamins, or minerals are not available at those times, development falters. Ill-timed exposures to medications (some anticonvulsants, antibiotics, and chemotherapeutic agents, for example), toxic agents in the environment (for instance, DDT, PCBs, mercury, lead), radiation, infectious agents, alcohol, and high levels of certain nutrients may also interrupt normal fetal development. Exposure to these insults during tissue and organ formation can result in miscarriage, malformations, or impaired physical and mental development of the fetus. The period of time during pregnancy when these exposures are most hazardous to the fetus is between implantation (approximately five days after conception) and eight weeks after conception.

Tissues and organs grow in size and weight after they have formed. This pattern of growth means that the major gains in fetal weight occur later in pregnancy. Once tissues and organs are formed, they are no longer vulnerable to insults that cause malformations. Insults occurring later in pregnancy, however, such as exposure to toxic substances and poor diets, may result in normally formed but undersized organs that do not function optimally.

Because there are so many factors that may affect tissue and organ development, it is almost always difficult to decide if a specific condition was responsible for a problem occurring in an individual newborn. Not every pregnancy is affected, or affected in the same ways, by exposure to harmful substances. In addition, many of the causes of abnormal fetal development are not known. Trying to isolate a single factor that may have disrupted fetal development or growth is usually an exercise in futility for any individual pregnancy.

Despite the susceptibility of the fetus during the first few months of pregnancy, most babies are born healthy and normal. Chances are excellent, however, that mothers intend to do the most and best they possibly can for their babies during pregnancy. The shared goal is an above-average baby, one that is as healthy and as well developed as possible. The outcome cannot be guaranteed, but it can be helped along by "growing the baby in the right oven."

Anticipating Changes in Your Body During Pregnancy

A woman's body goes through major changes to accommodate pregnancy. These changes occur throughout gestation and begin in earnest shortly after conception. Within the first weeks of pregnancy, hormones that support implantation of the embryo, growth of the uterus and placenta, and expansion of the mother's circulatory system are produced in abundance. This avalanche of hormones has side effects, however. It is likely responsible for the sore breasts, cramping, nausea, vomiting, and taste and smell changes experienced by many women very early in pregnancy. Around the third month, when nausea and vomiting often subside, fatigue may set in due to an expansion in blood volume. It takes from several weeks to over a month for a woman's body to get used to the higher volume of blood in the circulatory system.

During the first half of pregnancy, while the fetus is still quite small, a number of changes take place that cause the mother to store fat and nutrients. These stores are developed early so that they will be available to support major gains in fetal weight later. A direct consequence of the tendency to increase fat stores right away is that many women feel that they are becoming "fat" rather than pregnant. As pregnancy progresses, most women will stop storing fat and use up some of what they stored. Early gains in fat around the thighs, breasts, and trunk of the body have needlessly surprised and dismayed millions of women. Be aware: Adding fat stores is a pre-programmed phenomenon of the first half of pregnancy.

Appetite Changes

Most women find that their hunger frequency and food intake increases earlier in pregnancy than expected. We are biologically programmed to gain weight in advance of when we need it to support major gains in fetal weight. Weight gain may also be higher than expected in the early months of pregnancy because women may eat to relieve nausea and vomiting. Other times, food intake increases simply because women get really hungry often.

Weight gain early in pregnancy concerns many women. The worry that "I'm going to gain a ton if I keep eating like this" probably arises in almost everyone. The concern, however, may be misplaced. Changes in hunger and food intake during pregnancy normally come in spurts and plateaus. You may go through memorable periods of hunger and food intake one week and lose your high level of interest in eating the next. Expect that your level of hunger and food intake will vary somewhat during pregnancy, as will your rate of weight gain.

Most of the information presented about the normal course of hunger and food intake applies to pregnancies that are not complicated by restrictive eating practices, eating disorders, or exaggerated fears about weight gain. It is hard to find a woman who isn't concerned about gaining too much weight in pregnancy. However, a reasonable weight gain, which for most women should be somewhere between 25 and 35 pounds, is of critical importance to fetal development and growth. Much more is presented on the topic of weight gain and pregnancy in Chapter 7.

Preconceptional and Early Pregnancy Diet

A healthy diet to bring into pregnancy is characterized by the following:

- food intake that corresponds to the Food Guide Pyramid eating plan
- regular meals (no fasting or meal skipping)
- an intake of 400 µg (micrograms) (0.4 mg) folate per day
- no alcohol intake
- no overuse of dietary supplements
- enjoyment of food and mealtimes

These dietary basics apply to the first two months of pregnancy, too, but with one special consideration attached. Women should consume enough food to gain around 2 to 4 pounds during the first two months of pregnancy.

Following the Food Guide Pyramid

The cornerstone of a healthy diet is the selection of a variety of foods that together provide the level of energy and nutrients needed for maternal health and fetal development and growth. Because many components of food that promote health are not contained in supplements, healthy diets are based around food.

The best available guide for selecting a diet that promotes pre-conceptional and early pregnancy health is the Food Guide Pyramid (see Figure 2–1 in Chapter 2). This guide is much like the basic four (or five) food groups you probably learned about in school. This new revision of the basic food group guide is different in that it emphasizes building a healthy diet from the bottom of the food chain up. The Food Guide Pyramid provides a range of recommended number of servings for each food group. The lower number of servings is intended for people who have a lower need for calories, and the higher number of servings for individuals who are very physically active, growing, or are pregnant or breast-feeding. Serving sizes recommended are often smaller than food portion sizes.

The base of the Food Guide Pyramid consists of six to eleven servings each day of grain products such as bread, cereals, rice, and pasta. To emphasize their importance, vegetables (three to five servings each day of your favorites) and fruits (two to four servings) make up the next largest section of the Food Guide Pyramid. Milk and milk products, meats, and vegetarian protein foods take up a smaller space on the pyramid because we need fewer servings of them (two to three servings per day) than of grain products, vegetables, and fruits. For each of these food groups, the more "basic" the types of foods selected the better. For example, whole-grain products are preferred over refined grain products, and fresh meats are recommended over processed meats.

At the top of the Food Guide Pyramid is a small triangle that depicts the limited space in a healthy diet for fats, oils, and sweets. This does not mean that foods like butter, margarine, salad dressing, cookies, or desserts cannot be part of a healthy diet. It indicates that they should be a much smaller part of your diet than basic foods.

Do You Have a Healthy Diet?

Some women reading this information will already be consuming the recommended diet but may not know it. Others may be concerned about what they eat and want to identify specific changes they should make. The following exercise provides assurance that a healthy diet is being consumed or will pinpoint modifications needed.

To perform this evaluation, first think about your usual diet— what you customarily eat and drink. If your diet varies a good deal from day to day, pick several representative days for this exercise. Using the form provided in Table 4–1, write down everything you usually eat and drink starting with what you consumed after you awoke and recording your food and beverage intake throughout the day until bedtime.

Carefully estimate and record the amount of each food and beverage consumed. Next, compare your usual intake with that recommended in the Food Guide Pyramid. Table 4–2 provides a form. Make a mark in the appropriate food group for each serving of the food within that group you consumed in a day. Foods such as gravy, mayonnaise, margarine, chips, bacon, and rich desserts and candy go into the fats, oils, and sweets group. Foods like pretzels and popcorn, however, should go into the grain group. An abbreviated list of standard serving sizes is included in Table 4–2. Be sure to pay attention to the standard serving size. A cup of pasta is two servings, for example, and an ounce of cheese is two-thirds of a serving. If you need to, refer to the more complete list of standard serving sizes and foods included in each group given in Tables 2–8 and 2–9 in Chapter 2. If you consume mixed dishes such as pizza, stew, or burritos, break the dish into its major ingredients and record the amount of each ingredient consumed. Then assign each ingredient to its appropriate food group. Add up the number of servings you consumed in each food group and compare the results with the recommended number of servings. Voila! You have evaluated your diet.

If your results show that you are eating according to the Food Guide Pyramid, that is terrific!

If your diet is out of balance, identify specific foods you like within each food group that fell short. Then decide when you

Table 4–1 Usual Diet Recording Form

Time of Day	Day 1 What I Ate and Drank	Amount	Day 2 What I Ate and Drank	Amount
Example:				
Noon	Chef's salad:		Vegetarian lasagna:	
	Romaine	2 cups	pasta	1 cup
	turkey	1 ounce	tomato sauce	½ cup
	ham	1 ounce	zucchini	¼ cup
	cheese	1 ounce	cheese	1 ounce
	iced tea	1½ cups	milk	1 cup

Morning

Midmorning

Noon

Afternoon

Evening

Late evening

Table 4–2 Evaluating Your Preconception and Early Pregnancy Diet

Food Guide Pyramid group	Standard serving sizes	Recommended servings per day	Number of servings I had	Difference in servings
1. Bread, cereal, rice, and pasta	bread, 1 slice cereal, 1 cup hot cereal, ½ cup bagel, ½ rice or pasta, ½ cup tortilla, 1	6–11		
2. Vegetables	raw or cooked, ½ cup leafy, 1 cup juice, ¾ cup	3–5		
3. Fruits	fresh, 1 piece canned, ½ cup juice, ¾ cup	2–4		
4. Milk, yogurt, and cheese	milk, 1 cup soy milk, 1 cup yogurt, 1 cup cottage cheese, ½ cup cheese, 1½ ounces	2–3		
5. Meat, poultry, fish, dry beans, eggs, and nuts	meat, 3 ounces dried beans, ½ cup tofu, ½ cup eggs, 2 peanut butter, 4 tablespoons	2–3		
6. Fats, oils, and sweets	fats and oils, 2 teaspoons sweets, 1 ounce	limited		

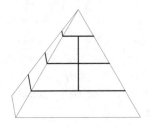

could eat those foods and what foods they should replace. Say, for example, you are short one serving from the milk, yogurt, and cheese group. Also assume you like frozen yogurt and skim milk and would enjoy eating them more often. You could decide to replace a snack such as cookies with a cup of frozen yogurt or substitute a glass of skim milk for a soft drink. If you would like to review a listing of foods within each basic food group to help get ideas for specific changes, refer to Table 2–9 in Chapter 2. You can also find recipes for healthy eating in Appendix A. The more specific plan you develop, and the more agreeable the plan is to you, the more likely it is that the change in dietary intake will be made and sustained.

What About Soda and Coffee?

Soft drinks sweetened with Nutrasweet appear to pose no risk during pregnancy. Diet sodas contribute little to a healthy diet, however.

You may want to limit coffee intake during pregnancy because of the association between intakes of over two cups of caffeinated coffee a day and miscarriage in some women. Neither coffee nor caffeine intake in pregnancy appears to be related to malformations.

Getting Enough Folate

In addition to eating a healthy diet, all women who may become pregnant should make sure they consume 400 µg (0.4 mg) of the vitamin folate from prior to conception through the first month after conception. Women who have had a baby with a neural tube defect, such as spina bifida, should take a supplement that contains a higher amount of folate prior to and early in pregnancy.

These recommendations of the U.S. Public Health Service stem from research results which show that low levels of folate intake within the first month of pregnancy cause about 70 percent of all cases of neural tube defects. Neural tube defects include spina bifida and brain malformations that develop within the first four weeks after conception. Because they develop so soon in pregnancy, the time to insure that your intake of folate is high enough is before you become pregnant.

How Do I Get Enough Folate?

You can get enough folate by consuming a 400 µg supplement of folic acid (a form of folate) or by consuming folate-fortified breakfast cereals. Most cold breakfast cereals are fortified with 100 µg of folic acid per serving and several cereals (Total and Product 19, for example) contain 400 µg of folic acid per serving. Check the nutrition information panel on the cereal package to confirm that the cereal you select is fortified. Daily consumption of a fortified cereal along with the variety of foods recommended in the Food Guide Pyramid will supply the needed amount of folate for most women. A list of food sources of folate is located in Appendix B.

It has recently become easier to obtain folate from the diet. Starting in January 1998, a regulation went into effect requiring that refined grained products be fortified with folic acid. Fortified breads, rice, crackers, pasta, and other refined grain products now provide about 40 µg of folic acid per serving.

The Importance of Regular Eating

If your usual eating pattern includes skipping meals or putting up with hunger until a convenient time to eat, this may be a good time to change it. Going without food for eight hours during the day may produce a less-than-optimal environment for early pregnancy. Eating three meals and, if needed, several snacks each day helps maintain an optimal glucose supply for the fetus. Glucose is the preferred source of energy for fetal development and growth. When we fast, blood levels of glucose drop somewhat and the fetus has to rely more heavily on fats as an energy source. Eating regular meals is also important later in pregnancy when the fetus gains most of its birth weight. The fetus needs increasing amounts of glucose as it grows larger, and that shortens the amount of time it takes for blood glucose levels in the mother to decline.

How Can I Change My Eating Pattern?

Changing your eating pattern is more easily recommended than done. Some women do not feel hungry often or can't even think about eating in the morning. The key to change in these circumstances is to do what you find acceptable. That may mean carrying around snacks, such as peanut butter and crackers, fruit, or granola, and eating "by the clock." It may mean drinking juice or milk in the morning rather than skipping breakfast altogether. As emphasized before, changes that are acceptable to you have the most staying power.

Taste and Smell Changes During Pregnancy

Approximately 50 percent of women notice changes in the way some foods taste and smell even before they are sure they are pregnant. These changes are so distinct that they can provide a strong clue that conception has occurred. Changes in the way certain foods taste and smell are considered normal early in pregnancy, and are predictive of a lower-than-average risk of miscarriage.

The types of foods that tend to taste worse in pregnancy vary, but many women develop a distaste for coffee, diet sodas, and alcohol-containing beverages. Sweet and salty foods are often reported to taste better, while the smell of foods frying makes some women queasy. Avoid foods which are offensive and, if possible, get someone else to cook if kitchen smells upset your stomach.

Specific food cravings are also known to occur in pregnancy. Some of these may be helpful, such as a craving for milk or fruit. Others, which lead to consumption of dirt, clay, or laundry starch, may be harmful.

Extreme changes in food preferences during pregnancy also occur but aren't considered normal. For example, if you make your husband or partner drive thirty miles in the middle of the night to get you watermelon, that's not a normal craving. A craving for lots of salty foods and water, excessive thirst, and a desire for orange juice, soft drinks, or other sugar-rich beverages after waking up may signal a problem with blood pressure or with glucose levels. These changes should be checked out by your health care provider.

The purpose of changes in food preferences during pregnancy does not appear to direct women toward a healthy selection of foods. There are no "maternal instincts" that improve food choices. Women have to make decisions about what to eat and what to avoid on their own.

Nausea and Vomiting During Early Pregnancy

Some 70 percent of women experience nausea within the first two months of pregnancy and about half experience vomiting. These symptoms generally begin within four weeks after conception and subside by nine or ten weeks. Nausea and vomiting last throughout pregnancy in 10 to 15 percent of women. Severe or prolonged nausea and vomiting are not considered normal and should be checked out by your health care provider.

Women who experience nausea or nausea and vomiting early in pregnancy are more than 30 percent less likely to miscarry than women who do not experience either nausea or vomiting. Increasing hormone levels that are thought to prompt nausea and vomiting may be responsible for the reduced risk of miscarriage.

It is preferable to "eat through" your nausea and vomiting rather than to lose weight. Additional information about nausea and vomiting in pregnancy and management advice are presented in Chapter 9.

Refraining from Alcohol Intake

Heavy alcohol intake (about five or more drinks per day) early in pregnancy is associated with miscarriage and the birth of infants who are malformed, small, and mentally impaired. Infants so affected are said to have *fetal alcohol syndrome,* or FAS. Regular drinking of smaller amounts of alcohol (a drink or more per day) early in pregnancy can also harm fetal development and growth but to a lesser extent. Excessive intake of alcohol later in pregnancy appears to impair growth and mental development but does not cause malformations. Adverse effects of an occasional drink in the second half of pregnancy appear to be rare. Since no amount of alcohol has been found to be absolutely safe during pregnancy, and to exclude the possibility of even small impairments to fetal development and growth, it is recommended that women do not drink alcohol if they may become pregnant or are pregnant.

Vitamin and Mineral Supplements

Should you take a vitamin and mineral supplement before and early in pregnancy? Several studies have shown a reduced risk of a number of malformations in babies born to women taking a multivitamin and mineral supplement before and early in pregnancy. On the other hand, studies indicate that large amounts of vitamin A (over 10,000 IU per day for months at a time) and vitamin D (intakes of over 1,000 IU regularly) may cause malformations. In a precautionary move in 1993, the American College of Obstetrics and Gynecology advised that vitamin A supplements not be used routinely during pregnancy and, if used, not more than 5,000 IU per day should be taken. It should be mentioned that supplements of beta-carotene, a precursor of vitamin A, have not been found to cause malformations.

Women are cautioned not to eat liver more often than weekly during early pregnancy because of its high vitamin A content. They are also advised not to use Retin A or Accutane medications for

Table 4–3 Recommended Allowances (RDAs): Preconception and the First Two Months of Pregnancy

Nutrient	RDA
Protein	46 g
Vitamin A	800 RE (4,000 IU)
Vitamin D	10 μg (400 IU)
Vitamin E	8 mg (24 IU)
Vitamin K	60 μg
Vitamin C	60 mg
Thiamin	1.1 mg
Riboflavin	1.3 mg
Niacin	15 mg NE
Vitamin B_6	1.6 mg
Folate	400 μg
Vitamin B_{12}	2 μg
Calcium	1,200 mg
Phosphorus	1,200 mg
Magnesium	280 mg
Iron	15 mg
Zinc	12 mg
Iodine	150 μg
Selenium	55 μg

Source: National Academy of Sciences, 1989.

acne and wrinkles because they are derived from vitamin A and their use early in pregnancy can cause miscarriage and malformations. It is best to stop use of these medications months in advance of conception.

Women who might become pregnant should not use high levels of vitamin and mineral supplements. Daily intakes of vitamins and minerals that correspond to the Recommended Dietary Allowances given in Table 4–3 are safe and may benefit some pregnancies.

Use of a multivitamin and mineral supplement is not routinely recommended for pregnancy. Iron supplements of 30 mg per day are recommended for all pregnant women starting after the twelfth week of pregnancy. Additional information about vitamin and mineral supplements and pregnancy is included in Chapter 6.

Other Considerations

Women who enter pregnancy with diabetes, hypertension, infectious disease, PKU (phenylketonuria—an inherited disorder), or who have had a previous baby with a congenital malformation or have a history of malformations in the family will most likely benefit from preconceptional care. Starting pregnancy in the best health possible can make a dramatic difference to maternal and fetal well-being.

5

The Right Diet
for Pregnancy

I am only one,
But still I am one.
I cannot do everything,
But still I can do something;
And because I cannot do everything
I will not refuse to do the something that I can do.

—E. E. Hale, 1822–1909

A s you have probably noticed, this book divides pregnancy into the early months (covered in the previous chapter) and the remaining months of pregnancy. This chapter addresses important aspects of nutrition during the last seven months of pregnancy, when fetal needs for energy and nutrients are primarily based on growth rather than on tissue and organ development. By the third month of pregnancy, most fetal tissues and organs have formed and are in the process of growing in size and complexity. A healthy diet is needed during these months primarily to support the growth of cells, maturation of the functional levels of organs, the development of the central nervous system, and the accumulation of fetal energy and the nutrient stores. During these seven months, fetal weight increases from about an ounce to approximately 8 pounds.

There are other components of good nutrition for pregnancy that don't fall under the heading of "diet." The topics of weight gain, vitamin and mineral supplements, exercise, nutritional aids for common problems of pregnancy, and nutrition for twin pregnancies will be covered in subsequent chapters.

Major changes take place within a woman's body during these months of gestation. The changes are so dramatic that they would be considered highly abnormal if it were not for pregnancy. The amount of blood in your circulatory system, your heart rate, appetite, food intake, and weight all increase significantly. Thanks to your expanded blood supply, you may notice that your hands and feet swell up a bit, especially late in pregnancy. Most women find that their bladders don't hold as much as they used to. Nausea and vomiting of early pregnancy may suddenly disappear in these months. Constipation and heartburn may, however, take their place. In addition, a number of other bothersome but normal changes can occur during pregnancy. People who presume the "healthy glow" of pregnancy overlies internal nirvana obviously haven't been pregnant!

This chapter presents the dietary ingredients of healthy infant outcomes and highlights nutrients of particular importance to pregnancy. You will be asked to evaluate your diet and offered suggestions for improving your dietary intake if changes are needed. A section on "fetal feeding" is included and explains how the fetus gets access to nutrients in your diet. The final portion of the chapter is devoted to answering questions pregnant women commonly ask about nutrition. If you have specific questions or concerns, check out this section. Hopefully, you will find the answers to your questions.

What Is a Healthy Diet for Pregnancy?

A woman's need for calories, protein, vitamins, minerals, and water all increase during pregnancy. With the exception of iron for many women, a careful selection of food can and should provide the additional calories and nutrients required. For healthy women, no special dietary supplements or foods are needed to insure adequate nutrition. What is needed is a diet that includes:

- sufficient calories to gain weight at an appropriate rate
- the assortment of foods recommended in the Food Guide Pyramid
- sufficient fluid (8 to 10 cups per day)
- enough high-fiber foods to prevent constipation

- no salt restriction
- no alcohol
- foods you enjoy and are consumed at pleasant mealtimes

Consuming Sufficient Calories to Gain Weight at the Appropriate Rate

No two women have exactly the same need for calories. That's because caloric need during pregnancy is based on an individual's physical activity level, current weight, muscle and fat mass, metabolic rate, and the stage of pregnancy. That makes it impossible to state with certainty a specific number of additional calories needed by individual pregnant women. The best way to judge the adequacy of caloric intake is by assessing weight gain.

When you consume more calories than you use up, you gain weight. When your caloric intake is lower than your body's need for calories, you lose it. In the best of all worlds, pregnant women would consume sufficient calories to consistently and gradually gain weight. The amount of weight gain that is right for pregnancy depends on prepregnancy weight and whether more than one baby is expected. (Specific information regarding weight gain is presented in Chapter 7.)

Appetite changes. If you are eating a healthy diet and gaining weight at the recommended rate, you really don't need to worry about calories. If your weight fluctuates a bit from day to day, you shouldn't worry about that either. Appetite and food intake levels during pregnancy come and go like the tide, only not as regularly. Good rates of weight gain often result when women eat when they are hungry and stop eating when they begin to feel full. Because this method doesn't work for all women, it may be necessary to monitor your weight gain in order to determine whether you are getting an adequate amount of calories.

Do You Have a Healthy Diet?

There are enough different aspects to a healthy diet in pregnancy to warrant a systematic evaluation rather than a brief, mental check. A systematic evaluation will allow you to identify specific changes in your diet that should be made or whether you're right on target. If you have read Chapter 4 on nutrition prior to and early in pregnancy, you'll already be familiar with this dietary evaluation method. Undertake this exercise even if you evaluated your diet earlier in pregnancy because weight gain and dietary requirements are different for this part of pregnancy.

Evaluation of your diet. To perform this evaluation, first think about your usual diet—what you customarily eat and drink. If your diet varies a good deal from day to day, pick several representative days for this exercise. Using the form provided in Table 5–1, write down everything you usually eat and drink starting with what you consume after you awake and then what you eat and drink throughout the day until bedtime. If it helps, carry a sheet of paper with you and record your food and beverage intake during the day or for several days.

Carefully estimate and record the amount of each food and beverage consumed. Serving size information on food package labels can help you identify food amounts. Next, compare your usual intake with that recommended in the Food Guide Pyramid. Table 5–2 provides a form for recording this information.

Make a mark in the appropriate food group for each serving of the food you consumed in a day. Foods such as gravy, mayonnaise, margarine, chips, bacon, and rich desserts and candy go into the fats, oils, and sweets group. Refer to Table 2–9 in Chapter 2 for additional information about the food groups. Be sure to pay attention to standard serving sizes—they are often smaller than you may guess. If you need to, refer to the more complete list of standard serving sizes given in Table 2–8. If you consume mixed dishes such as pizza, stew, or burritos, break the dish into its major ingredients and record the amount of each ingredient consumed. Then assign each ingredient to its appropriate food group. Add up the number of servings you consumed in each food group and compare the results with the recommended number of servings. You've done it! You have evaluated your pregnancy diet.

If your results show that you are eating according to the Food Guide Pyramid and you are gaining weight at an appropriate

Table 5–1 Usual Diet Recording Form

Time of Day	DAY 1		DAY 2	
	What I Ate and Drank	**Amount**	**What I Ate and Drank**	**Amount**
Example:				
Noon	Chef's salad:		Vegetarian lasagna:	
	Romaine	2 cups	pasta	1 cup
	turkey	1 ounce	tomato sauce	½ cup
	ham	1 ounce	zucchini	¼ cup
	cheese	1 ounce	cheese	1 ounce
	iced tea	1½ cups	milk	1 cup
Morning				
Midmorning				
Noon				
Afternoon				
Evening				
Late evening				

Table 5–2 Evaluating Your Pregnancy Diet

Food Guide Pyramid group	Standard serving sizes	Recommended servings per day	Number of servings I had	Difference in servings
1. Bread, cereal, rice, and pasta	bread, 1 slice cereal, 1 cup hot cereal, ½ cup bagel, ½ rice or pasta, ½ cup tortilla, 1	6–11		
2. Vegetables	raw or cooked, ½ cup leafy, 1 cup juice, ¾ cup	3–5		
3. Fruits	fresh, 1 piece canned, ½ cup juice, ¾ cup	2–4		
4. Milk, yogurt, and cheese	milk, 1 cup soy milk, 1 cup yogurt, 1 cup cottage cheese, ½ cup cheese, 1½ ounces	3		
5. Meat, poultry, fish, dry beans, eggs, and nuts	meat, 3 ounces dried beans, ½ cup tofu, ½ cup eggs, 2 peanut butter, 4 tablespoons	2–3		
6. Fats, oils, and sweets	fats and oils, 2 teaspoons sweets, 1 ounce	limited		

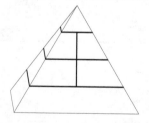

pace, nice going. Skip the next paragraph while patting yourself on the back.

If your diet is out of balance or your weight gain is off track, think about what changes could be made. To modify your diet, identify specific foods you like within each food group that fell short. Then decide when you could eat those foods and, if your diet contains too many servings of particular food groups, which foods they should replace. For example, assume you are one serving short on vegetables. Also assume that you like carrot sticks and cherry tomatoes and would enjoy eating them more often. You could decide to replace a snack such as a candy bar with a cup of carrot sticks and cherry tomatoes. If you would like to review a listing of foods within each basic food group to help get ideas for specific changes, refer to Table 2–9 in Chapter 2. As a reminder, you can find recipes for healthy eating in Appendix A. If your weight gain is too low, a plan for adding foods at mealtimes or for snacking more often should be developed. If it is too high, decide which foods or portion sizes can be reduced. The more specific plan you develop, and the more acceptable the plan is to you, the more likely it is that the change in dietary intake will be made and sustained.

Getting Enough Fluids

Most women need about eight to ten cups of fluid (or 64 to 80 ounces) daily during pregnancy. This amount of fluid is usually obtained from beverages and foods that are part of the regular diet. Women tend to consume as much fluid as they need because the body has internal thirst mechanisms that signal "I'm thirsty" when the body is running short on water. These internal mechanisms, however, may not make individuals thirsty enough when the need for water is high. Pregnant women who are exposed to hot, humid climates may fail to consume enough fluid if they depend on the "I'm thirsty" internal signal. Getting enough fluids is also a concern for women who experience vomiting in pregnancy. In these situations, women are urged to drink water regularly even if they don't feel thirsty. It will help keep your energy level up and the chances of developing dehydration down.

Consuming Enough High-Fiber Foods

Constipation is a common problem in pregnancy that can often be prevented by high-fiber diets. High-fiber foods are generally good sources of a variety of nutrients, so they are good to eat even if constipation isn't a problem.

How much fiber is enough to prevent constipation? Generally 25 grams a day along with plenty of water is sufficient. Where do you get fiber? Table 2–2 in Chapter 2 lists food sources of fiber. Choose the sources you like and can fit into your diet. Powdered, supplemental fiber you can buy in many pharmacies and grocery stores also works. (Fiber pills are not recommended because of their size.) If you use powdered fiber, follow the directions on the container. Individuals vary a good deal in their sensitivity to fiber. An overdose may cause diarrhea, and if too little water is consumed, fiber can be constipating. Water allows fiber to swell and create the bulk that stimulates the movement of waste products along the intestinal tract. You know you have consumed the right amount of fiber when your stools are soft and well formed.

No Salt Restriction

The American College of Obstetrics and Gynecology advises that restricting salt intake during pregnancy is not beneficial and may be harmful. Women should not restrict salt or sodium intake during pregnancy. Women who enter pregnancy with hypertension may need to watch their salt and sodium intake carefully. For these women, specific recommendations on salt and sodium intake should be obtained from their health care providers.

No Alcohol

It is recommended that pregnant women refrain from drinking alcohol-containing beverages because alcohol may harm the fetus. If you would like additional information about this topic, refer to Chapter 4.

Enjoy Foods You Like

We have something to learn from the Japanese Dietary Guidelines. The last guideline states: "Make all activities pertaining to food and eating pleasurable ones." All-too-busy Americans sometimes forget about the joy of eating good food with family and friends. Take the time to devote your attention to the foods you eat and to enjoy mealtimes. Bon appetit!

Key Nutrients for Pregnancy

It is important to consume enough of every nutrient required during pregnancy. Certain nutrients, however, deserve a spotlight because they are most likely to be present in low amounts in the diets of pregnant women. You will notice that protein is not included in the nutrients highlighted. That is because American women rarely lack protein in their diets. If you think your intake of protein or any of the nutrients presented is low, refer to Tables 2–2 to 2–5 and Appendix B and compare your intake of good food sources of the nutrients in question to foods listed in the table. Use the RDAs (Recommended Dietary Allowances) for pregnancy listed in Table 5–3 as a rough guide of the amount of nutrients you should consume.

The information presented on key nutrients does not address nutrient overdoses. That is because overdoses of vitamins and minerals result from the overuse of supplements nearly 100 percent of the time. Cautions regarding the excessive use of supplements are discussed in Chapter 6.

Key Nutrient #1: Folate

Folate has gained prominence as a vitamin you need in ample amounts prior to and very early in pregnancy. Your need for extra folate continues throughout the rest of pregnancy and many women do not consume enough of it. Consumption of an adequate amount of folate (400 µg or 0.4 mg per day) helps prevent the development of certain types of anemia and promotes the growth of fetal tissues and organs. It is needed for the formation of protein tissues in both the mother and the fetus.

Table 5–3 Recommended Allowances (RDAs) for Pregnancy

Nutrient	RDA
Protein	60 g
Vitamin A	800 RE (4,000 IU)
Vitamin D	10 µg (400 IU)
Vitamin E	8 mg (24 IU)
Vitamin K	65 µg
Vitamin C	70 mg
Thiamin	1.5 mg
Riboflavin	1.6 mg
Niacin	17 mg NE
Vitamin B_6	2.2 mg
Folate	400 µg
Vitamin B_{12}	2.2 µg
Calcium	1,200 mg
Phosphorus	1,200 mg
Magnesium	320 mg
Iron	30 mg
Zinc	15 mg
Iodine	175 µg
Selenium	65 µg

Source: National Academy of Sciences, 1989.

Folate means *foliage.* It was first discovered in spinach and is found in most types of leafy green vegetables. However, folate is present in a variety of other foods we don't think of as being leafy and green. These foods include broccoli, oranges, bananas, milk, and dried beans. Vegetables and fruits provide an average of 42 µg folate per serving. Breakfast cereals are generally fortified with folic acid, a form of folate that is highly absorbable. Refined grain products such as bread, grits, white rice, crackers, and pasta are, by law, fortified with folic acid. Each serving of these grain products provides approximately 40 µg of folic acid per serving. So, if you consume five servings of fruits and vegetables daily and six servings of refined grain products, your total folate intake will likely be at least 400 µg, or the recommended amount.

Key Nutrient #2: Vitamin D

Women who consume three or more cups daily of milk or soy milk fortified with vitamin D, or receive sufficient exposure to sunshine (one to two hours per week in the summer) likely receive sufficient vitamin D for pregnancy. Women with dark skin need two hours or more per week of sunshine to produce sufficient vitamin D. Interestingly, our bodies can make vitamin D when skin is directly exposed to sunshine. Because most of our vitamin D supply comes from milk and the sun, women who don't drink milk or whose skin isn't exposed to direct sunshine due to cold climates, sunscreen use, or clothing that covers most of the body are at risk of poor vitamin D levels. Exposing skin to the weak rays of the sun during the winter in cold climates doesn't produce much, if any, vitamin D. (The fact that vitamin D doesn't form when skin is exposed to the weak rays of the sun in northern climates during the winter was recently reported. A professor in Boston sent several scantily clad graduate students to a rooftop to sunbathe for awhile in the middle of winter. The results: all the students got was cold. The sunlight was too weak to produce any vitamin D whatsoever in their skin.) Rickets, the vitamin D deficiency disease, is periodically reported in infants whose mothers habitually cover almost all their skin with clothing and who do not drink milk. Of all the dairy products, only milk is fortified with vitamin D in the United States.

Some breakfast cereals are fortified with 40 IU vitamin D per serving so that they can contribute to vitamin D intake. Because many breakfast cereals are not fortified with vitamin D, you really have to check the label to be sure that vitamin D has been added. An intake of 400 IU of vitamin D per day is recommended for pregnancy.

Vitamin D supports fetal growth, the calcification of bone (or the addition of calcium to bone), and tooth and enamel formation. Enough is as good as a feast, however. Intakes of vitamin D from foods and supplements should not exceed 1,000 IU per day on a regular basis.

Key Nutrient #3: Iron

Women have a high need for iron during pregnancy because it is used to form hemoglobin in red blood cells and for fetal growth. That is why the RDA for iron in pregnancy is a whopping 30 mg. Most women consume less than half that amount, and it is common for women to conceive without sufficient stores to cover the iron cost of pregnancy. Consequently, iron supplements are recommended for all pregnant women.

It is possible for women to get enough iron from their diets, but it takes a careful selection of food. One of the easiest ways to obtain iron from the diet is to consume a highly fortified breakfast cereal (such as Product 19 or Total). These cereals are fortified with 18 mg of iron per serving. Other breakfast cereals are fortified with 4 or 5 mg of iron per serving. The absorption of iron from cereals can be doubled or tripled if consumed with a source of vitamin C such as orange or grapefruit juice. Absorption of iron from plant foods such as kale, turnip greens, collard greens, asparagus, black-eyed peas, dried beans, and spinach is also increased substantially if foods high in vitamin C are consumed at the same meal. Appendix B lists good food sources of iron and vitamin C. It should be pointed out that the RDA for iron is based on iron intake, and not the amount of iron absorbed.

Absorption of iron from meats is more complete than that from plants. On average, a 3-ounce serving of red meat (about the size of a deck of cards) supplies 3 mg of iron, and a 3-ounce serving of fish or poultry, 1 mg of iron. Liver is an excellent source of iron (providing 7.5 mg per 3 ounces), but because it contains very high amounts of vitamin A, it should be consumed no more than once weekly.

Cast-iron pans are a good source of iron because some of the iron in the pan is absorbed by the food during cooking. Although it is hard to say how much iron you get from the pan, it is likely to be several milligrams or more per serving of food cooked for ten to fifteen minutes. Acidic foods like tomatoes and applesauce leach more iron from iron pans than do foods such as potatoes or eggs.

If you're a newcomer to cast-iron pans, make sure you "season" them with heat and a light coating of vegetable oil before you use them. Iron pans are cleaned by scrubbing them in hot water (no soap) and then heating them on the stove. A light coating of vegetable oil applied to the bottom of the pan before use keeps foods from sticking when they are cooked. Perhaps a friend or relative could give you advice on seasoning new iron pans to perfection. It's becoming a lost art.

Key Nutrient #4: Zinc

The RDA for zinc during pregnancy is 15 mg, and most women consume 10 to 12 mg per day during pregnancy. Zinc and iron are found in many of the same foods (meats, fortified breakfast cereals, and dried beans). Adequate zinc levels in pregnancy help women resist infectious diseases, may help prevent abnormally long labor, and support fetal growth.

Key Nutrient #5: Calcium

Calcium is a key nutrient for women who don't consume three or more servings per day of dairy products or calcium-fortified soy milk; it is difficult to get the recommended 1,200 mg per day without using these foods. Appendix B provides a list of food sources that may be helpful in identifying foods you could eat to meet your need for calcium.

A lack of calcium in the mother's diet doesn't jeopardize fetal bone growth as does inadequate levels of vitamin D. If a woman's intake of calcium is low, calcium from the mother's bones will be used to meet fetal needs for calcium. There is evidence that low calcium intake may be involved in the development of hypertension during pregnancy.

Key Nutrient #6: Vitamin C

Women who smoke need more vitamin C than women who don't. Smokers should consume around 200 mg of vitamin C per day, whereas nonsmokers need 70 mg daily. You can obtain 200 mg by eating three to four servings of food sources of vitamin C daily such as kiwi fruit, oranges, orange juice, cantaloupe, grapefruit, grapefruit juice, green pepper, cauliflower, broccoli, and brussels sprouts. It would, of course, be preferable to reduce the need for vitamin C by calling a halt to smoking.

There are other advantages to consuming vitamin C–rich foods. These foods tend to contain other beneficial substances that appear to reduce the risk of infection and certain diseases. The benefits of consuming a variety of food sources of vitamin C may be due to the vitamin C as well as to other substances found in vitamin C–rich foods.

Fetal Feeding

Only well-nourished women are in a position to optimally nourish a fetus. That is because when you eat, the nutrients consumed in foods do not go directly to the fetus. The body processes the nutrients by first changing them into forms the body can use. After nutrients are processed by the body and made available for use, the mother's needs for them are generally met first. For example, if a woman's iron stores are low or if too little vitamin D is available, the incoming supply of iron or vitamin D will be first used to meet the mother's needs. When the mother's need for iron or vitamin D is met, the placenta gets priority on the available nutrient supply. When the placenta has a sufficient supply of nutrients to grow and function normally, then the fetus is given access to available nutrients. The bottom line is that the fetus does not get "first dibs" on nutrients supplied by the mother's diet. The priority system of favoring the mother's nutrient supply over that of a fetus makes sense biologically. Mother Nature is favoring the health of the reproducer. For optimal fetal growth, diets during pregnancy must meet the needs of both the mother and the fetus.

Commonly Asked Questions About Diet and Pregnancy

This section addresses many of the questions commonly asked by pregnant women. The questions are divided into four categories:

- general diet
- foods to eat or avoid
- appetite and food cravings
- diet and changes in a woman's body

No doubt some of the questions addressed haven't occurred to you. Reading this section may answer them before you need to ask.

General Diet

Q. *How much should I eat during pregnancy?*

A. Enough to gain weight at the appropriate rate (see Chapter 7). The amount of food a woman should consume during pregnancy varies by her level of physical activity and other factors. There is no one amount of weight to gain that's right for everyone. If you are concerned, the best way to judge whether you are eating enough, or too much, is to monitor your weight gain using the information provided in Chapter 7.

Q. *How do I know if I'm eating enough for the baby?*

A. You can usually know by your weight gain. If your weight gain is on target (see Chapter 7), you most likely are eating enough for the baby.

Sometimes women will gain a good deal of weight (2 or more pounds in a week) while they are not eating that much. The gain may be due to water retention. Women who are retaining water may have swelling, or *edema,* in their lower legs and hands. In this case, you can't count on your weight as being a good indicator of whether you are eating enough or too much. Eating basic foods to satisfy your appetite, or at least not restricting your food intake, may be your best guide in this situation.

A large, unexpected gain in weight can signal a problem with blood pressure. Make sure you let your health care provider know if this occurs.

Q. *I was heavy before pregnancy. Do I need to eat as much as other women?*

A. You need to eat enough to maintain a gradual gain in weight. If you started pregnancy weighing more than 130 percent of average weight for height (see Table 3–1 in Chapter 3), you should try to gain around ½ pound per week. Pregnancy is not the time to lose weight, no matter what your prepregnancy weight was.

Q. *Do I need to eat special foods?*

A. No. You just need to eat an adequate and well-balanced diet that consists of a wide variety of nutritious foods.

Q. *I'm a vegan. Anything special I should do?*

A. A vegan diet can still be a healthy one during pregnancy. It is prudent, however, to assess your intake of vitamin B_{12}, vitamin D, calcium, iron, and zinc; and to monitor your weight gain. The table of the RDAs for pregnancy (Table 5–1), and the food sources of nutrients table in Chapter 2, can help you assess your intake of these key nutrients. Information in Chapter 7 addresses the question, "How much weight should I gain?" Fortified soy milk and breakfast cereals are usually good sources of these key nutrients. You should check the nutrition information labels on soy milk and cereal packages to be sure, however. A multivitamin and mineral supplement can be used if needed. Unless the diagnosis of a specific nutrient deficiency has been made, it is best to use supplements that contain no more than 100 percent of the RDA for pregnancy.

Protein intake of vegans is likely adequate if diets follow the Food Guide Pyramid recommendations.

Q. *Won't the baby just take what it needs from me, regardless of what I eat?*

A. The fetus does not act like a parasite. What you eat is important. The mother's diet and nutrient stores need to be adequate to meet her own needs as well as those of the growing fetus. For most nutrients, if the available supply of energy or nutrient is low, it's the mother who gets "first dibs" on the available supply. This built-in system for energy and nutrient allocation during pregnancy fosters the well-being of the mother over that of the fetus, thereby promoting the health of the reproducer first. Infants have been born with various vitamin deficiency diseases to women who show no signs of deficiency.

Q. *Doesn't the placenta protect the baby from harmful things that may be in the mother's diet?*

A. To some extent, yes. But the placenta cannot protect the fetus from all things harmful. Alcohol and high levels of intake of supplements, for example, are transferred to and may harm the fetus. You can't count on the placenta to provide 100 percent protection against harmful components of the diet.

Q. *Won't my body tell me what foods to eat during pregnancy?*

A. There is no inner voice that directs women to a nutritious diet during pregnancy. Women make those decisions based on years of learning experiences involving foods.

Q. *How much protein do I need?*

A. According to the RDAs, you need 60 grams of protein per day. If you're a vegan, you should aim for 70 to 80 grams. Protein intakes of 70 to 80 grams per day are common among pregnant women in America and represent a healthy level of intake.

You can estimate how much protein is in your diet by undertaking the evaluation described in the first paragraph under the "Key Nutrients for Pregnancy" section of this chapter.

Q. *Should I watch my fat intake?*

A. Pregnancy does not appear to be the time to go on a low-fat diet. A low-fat diet may interfere with getting enough calories and may deprive the fetus of certain types of fats that are needed for fetal development.

Q. *How much water should I drink?*

A. "Drink to thirst" is the general advice. Specific recommendations depend on your situation. Unless you live in a warm, humid climate, an intake of eight to ten cups of fluids each day from water, fruit juice, milk, and other beverages, as well as foods, is adequate. Women exposed to heat and humidity may need more than ten cups of fluid each day. Sufficient fluid should be consumed to replace that lost in sweat. That may mean drinking water or other fluids regularly whether you feel thirsty or not.

Q. *I'm not eating that much more than I did before pregnancy, yet I'm gaining weight. How can that happen?*

A. That often happens in pregnancy. It is probably due to a decrease in physical activity. Many women reduce their levels of physical activity during pregnancy while not changing their food intake very much. Calories saved from a lower expenditure of energy on physical activity can contribute to weight gain.

Unexpected increases in weight of over 2 pounds a week may mean that you are retaining water. Weight gain that catches you by surprise should be discussed with your health care provider.

Q. *Should I ask for a referral to, or make an appointment with, a dietitian/ nutritionist during pregnancy?*

A. The answer is "yes" for women who:

- doubt that the information or advice they have been given about nutrition is accurate
- have been given insufficient information about a nutritional concern to be able to make the appropriate change
- have gestational diabetes or entered pregnancy with a disorder such as PKU, chronic renal disease, diabetes, or an eating disorder; have problems gaining weight or eating a healthy diet; or are on a restrictive diet.

Perinatal dietitians/nutritionists specialize in pregnancy and are your best resource. Many managed care organizations have dietitians/nutritionists on staff and most insurance companies will reimburse the costs for services of a bona fide dietitian/nutritionist with a doctor's referral or sometimes upon a patient's request. If there is a question about coverage, call your insurance provider. If you don't have medical insurance, call your local health department and ask to speak with a nutritionist who knows about pregnancy.

Q. *Our family has run into tough times and we don't have enough money for food. Can we get help?*

A. Yes. The first step is to call your local health department and ask about food and nutrition assistance programs. Many communities have food pantries, free meal programs, Second Harvest programs, and other types of assistance available. If your yearly household income is low (less than about $19,600 for a family of two), you may be eligible for the "WIC" program. This food and nutrition education program is specifically designed for low-income pregnant women and children at nutritional risk.

Q. *Is it okay to drink or eat during labor?*

A. It depends on who you ask. Some health care providers insist that women should not eat or drink during labor, while others think it's a myth. The primary reason for not allowing fluids and food during labor is related to the possible use of general anesthesia. If general anesthesia is used for a surgical delivery, vomiting may occur and some of the contents of the stomach may be inhaled into the lungs. That can cause serious problems. On the other hand, some health care providers allow women to drink fluids or to eat light foods during labor if the likelihood is extremely low that general anesthesia will be used. They believe that allowing fluid and food helps keep the woman hydrated and may help prevent fatigue.

Going through the active part of labor on a full stomach is probably like eating a big meal right before you swim the English Channel; it is not a good idea.

Foods to Eat or Avoid

Q. *Do I have to eat meat?*

A. No. You can get the nutrients you need for pregnancy from foods other than meat. As recommended for all pregnant women, you should check out your diet to make sure you are eating an appropriate assortment of foods. If your diet follows the Food Guide Pyramid recommendations, you can have a healthy diet without eating meat.

Q. *Do I have to drink milk?*

A. No. But you do need to make sure you get enough calcium and vitamin D. Milk is a nutrient-dense food that is hard to replace in the diet. If you can drink milk, you should. It is an excellent source of calcium and vitamin D. Low-fat chocolate milk is a good choice for women who prefer it over regular milk.

Consuming four servings of cheese, yogurt, cottage cheese, or fortified soy milk along with the other components of a healthy diet should meet your needs for calcium. However, because vitamin D is only found in milk and not other dairy products, you may have to get at least some of your vitamin D from exposing your skin to sunshine or from a supplement.

Q. *Dairy products give me gas and cramps so I don't eat them. What other foods can I eat to get enough calcium?*
A. You may have lactose intolerance. If so, you can consume low-lactose milk and probably yogurt, or you can take a lactase pill before you eat dairy products; however, lactase pills tend to be quite expensive.

Many, but not all, people with lactose intolerance can eat small amounts of dairy products with few or no side effects. You may be able to drink a cup or a half-cup of milk, or eat an ounce of cheese at a meal and feel no discomfort. Many types of yogurt contain little lactose and are easily digested. Low- and no-lactose milks are widely available. If you have trouble tolerating a low-lactose milk, you should try a no-lactose product. Low-lactose and no-lactose milk tends to taste a bit sweeter than regular milk.

Another reason some people don't tolerate dairy products well is an allergy to cow's milk protein. This condition is rare in adults but if it exists, substituting no-lactose milk for regular milk won't relieve the unpleasant symptoms. Supplements containing 600 mg calcium and 200 IU vitamin D may be the best alternative if you are allergic to milk and dairy products.

Q. *Do spicy foods hurt the baby?*
A. No. Components of spicy foods that end up in the mother's blood are not harmful to the fetus.

Q. *Should I avoid food additives while I'm pregnant?*
A. Food additives that weren't a problem before you conceived should not become one during pregnancy. In general, food additives are considered safe.

Q. *Are caffeinated soft drinks a problem?*
A. They don't appear to be a problem for pregnant women.

Q. *Is it okay to drink diet sodas if you are pregnant?*
A. They appear to be safe.

Q. *Is it okay to drink herbal teas?*

A. That's a good question that doesn't have a satisfactory answer. It is not known which herbal teas are safe to consume and which should be avoided in pregnancy. Consequently, consumption of herbal teas cannot be recommended in pregnancy.

Q. *I'm over halfway through my pregnancy. Will an occasional drink of wine or beer hurt the baby?*

A. Probably not . . . but it is still best not to drink. It appears that a drink or two a week from midpregnancy on may not damage the fetus in an easily noticeable way. However, harmful effects cannot be ruled out. One study found that as little as one drink a day in pregnancy was related to attention deficit disorder in children at age fourteen. When a pregnant woman has a drink, so does her fetus. Alcohol is rapidly transported from the mother's blood to that of the fetus. To be on the safe side, it is better not to drink at all during pregnancy.

Q. *Will it harm my baby if I drink coffee during pregnancy?*

A. Coffee consumption in the first two months of pregnancy is weakly related to the risk of miscarriage. However, drinking coffee after the first two months does not appear to harm the baby and drinking several cups of coffee per day is considered safe. There is some question as to whether high coffee intakes (seven or more cups per day), or the consumption of several cups of very strong coffee a day may reduce fetal growth somewhat. Coffee intake has not been associated with the development of malformations in the baby nor with health or behavioral problems later in childhood.

Q. *I don't want to become anemic but I don't like taking my iron pills. Are there foods I can eat that will prevent anemia?*

A. Yes, there are. The requirement for iron increases a good deal in pregnancy, however, and it may be difficult to get enough iron without taking a supplement. Women who enter pregnancy with a good supply of stored iron and who consume foods high in iron and vitamin C maintain better iron levels than women who conceive with low iron stores and take in few sources of iron and vitamin C. If iron levels become low, an iron supplement in a dose that can be easily tolerated should be used. Low doses of iron (30 mg per day) are generally much better tolerated than are higher doses.

Q. *I've heard some fish may be contaminated with environmental toxins. Is eating fish a problem during pregnancy?*

A. Only if the fish come from contaminated waters. Avoid eating fish caught in rivers posted as contaminated. You can assume that fish purchased in seafood markets and grocery stores is safe.

Q. *Are certain vegetables, like strong-tasting ones, bad for your baby?*

A. Claims that certain vegetables such as broccoli, brussels sprouts, cabbage, garlic, and cauliflower make women nauseous or harm their fetuses have not been shown to be true. Eat the variety of vegetables you like. They really are good for you and the baby.

Q. *Should I cut back on salt?*

A. Pregnant women in general should not restrict their salt intake.

The practice of routinely restricting the salt intake of pregnant women hasn't completely faded away in this and other countries, although it is not a good idea. Salt restriction may actually be harmful and is associated with a poorer-quality diet, reduced weight gain, and the birth of underweight infants. There is no evidence that salt restriction helps reduce high blood pressure that develops in pregnancy. Salt restriction may actually aggravate problems with blood pressure. Although pregnant women should not eat salt to excess, it should be consumed "to taste." Many women find that their desire for salt and salty foods increases somewhat during pregnancy. That is a normal change.

Women entering pregnancy with hypertension that was partially controlled by a salt-restricted diet should maintain a diet that is slightly less restrictive of salt than the prepregnancy one. That is because pregnant women have an increased need for sodium. Women with preexisting hypertension should work closely with their doctors and a dietitian/nutritionist on the control of their blood pressure during and after pregnancy.

Appetite and Food Cravings

Q. *My appetite isn't that good. What can I do about it?*

A. If you're not gaining weight and your appetite has been poor for more than a week, you may have to eat by the clock rather than by your appetite. That means eating meals at regular times and carrying around snacks. Small, frequent meals sometimes go down easier than large ones in women with poor appetite.

If the poor appetite is due to nausea or vomiting during pregnancy, go to Chapter 9 for specific advice.

Q. *The other morning at breakfast I ate six big pancakes. They tasted delicious but I'm usually stuffed after two. What's happening?*

A. You have entered the "hunger zone." Periods of above-average hunger and food intake are characteristic of periods of growth. You shouldn't worry too much about it. Hunger periods come and go.

Q. *Ever since I became pregnant I've been craving certain foods. My friends says it's all in my head. These cravings are normal, right?*

A. Yes, they are normal as long as they are not too weird (like craving the smell of Comet cleanser or gasoline). Taste and food preferences normally change somewhat during pregnancy.

Q. *Shortly after I became pregnant I developed a strong craving for a particular type of clay. Will it hurt my baby if I sometimes eat it?*

A. It may. Some women find the smell and taste of a specific type of clay irresistible in pregnancy. Other women are attracted to dry laundry starch, dirt, or other substances that are not thought of as being food. Consumption of clay or dirt may clog up the intestines or cause infection or parasitic infestation of the intestinal tract. If the clay or dirt settles the stomach, there are medicines that can be more safely used. Some women find dried powdered milk is a good substitute for dry laundry starch.

Q. *I've been craving ice cubes and ice chips lately and can't seem to stop crunching on them. What's up?*

A. You may have iron deficiency anemia. Have your health care provider check for it.

Ice eating is often, but not always, associated with iron deficiency anemia. It's not known why the two conditions occur together.

Q. *Will the baby let me know when it's time to eat?*

A. No. Your body sets off the hunger alarm.

Q. *Will it hurt the baby if I don't eat the foods I'm craving?*

A. Food cravings during pregnancy do not appear to be based on the needs of the fetus. Consequently, you shouldn't feel compelled to eat the specific foods you crave.

Q. *Constipation has recently become a problem. What can I do about it?*

A. Eat more fiber and drink more water. If you are not physically active, some exercise may also help.

Constipation can usually be prevented if you regularly consume 25 grams of fiber a day along with plenty of fluids. Table 2–2 in Chapter 2 lists food sources of fiber. High-fiber breakfast cereals and supplemental fiber, such as a daily teaspoon or two of bran or Metamucil or a similar product mixed with water or juice, may be particularly helpful. Additional advice about getting enough fiber is given in Chapter 2.

Q. *What can I do about heartburn?*

A. Eat small frequent meals and avoid having your head lower than your stomach. If iron or other supplements seem to aggravate the heartburn, stop the supplements for a few days or take them less often and see if that helps. If going off the supplements helps, seek your health care provider's advice on whether you should discontinue them. Your health care provider may recommend antacid tablets. Read more about the prevention of heartburn in Chapter 9.

Diet and Changes in a Woman's Body

Q. *My hemoglobin dropped two points over the last two months. Is that normal?*

A. A drop in hemoglobin during pregnancy is normal—if it doesn't drop too far.

A drop in hemoglobin is generally considered to be a good sign because it indicates that the volume of blood in your circulatory system is increasing. A healthy increase in blood volume is associated with good rates of fetal growth. Women are not considered to have iron deficiency anemia until their hemoglobin drops below 10.5 g/dl (grams per deciliter) in the second trimester, or below 11.0 g/dl in the third trimester. Hemoglobins that don't fall a bit, or that are high, are more of a cause for concern than are hemoglobins that drop somewhat. A rising hemoglobin, unless it is in response to iron supplements taken for anemia, may indicate that blood volume is not expanding appropriately.

Q. *I'm seven months pregnant and had my blood tested for cholesterol and triglycerides at a health fair. I couldn't believe how high they were! Do I need to go on a special diet to lower my levels of cholesterol and triglycerides?*

A. No special diet is indicated.

Cholesterol and triglycerides normally increase substantially in pregnancy, especially during the third trimester. The fetus has a high need for cholesterol as it is required to form nervous tissue and cell membranes. Triglycerides go up because they are a source of energy for the fetus. If you are concerned, have your blood tested again after pregnancy or several months after you have weaned your baby if you breast-feed.

A carefully chosen diet provides the best insurance that you are getting the assortment and amount of nutrients needed for pregnancy. Nonetheless, vitamins and minerals are often taken to "supplement" the diet in pregnancy. Reasons for using supplements, and cautions about their use, are discussed in the next chapter.

6

Vitamin and Mineral Supplements

Enough is as good as a feast.

—Mary Poppins

Two of the most powerful words in our nutrition vocabulary are vitamins and minerals. They are the health-giving, life-sustaining, disease-preventing elements of food. The general view of vitamins and minerals is so positive that we tend to believe they cannot be harmful; that the more we consume, the better. This view of vitamins and minerals may be the leading reason why supplements tend to be overused during pregnancy.

It has become almost expected that a health care provider will prescribe a multivitamin and mineral supplement as soon as pregnancy is confirmed. If not, the quality of care may be questioned. The expectation of receiving such a supplement has become so ingrained that it is proving difficult to change, even though a better approach is known and recommended.

The superior way of ensuring adequate vitamin and mineral intake in pregnancy is through diet and not supplements. There are several reasons for this. First, not all of the nutrients needed for optimal fetal development and growth are available in supplements. Foods contain many substances in addition to vitamins and minerals that promote development, growth, and health. Vitamin and mineral supplements should also not be viewed as insurance against harms caused by poor diets. They are Band-Aids that may temporarily help heal wounds caused by a poor selection of foods, but any benefits last only as long as the supplements do. Good nutrition should be for life and not just for the period of pregnancy.

A final reason caution is called for regarding the use of vitamin and mineral supplements in pregnancy is that too much of a good thing can be harmful. Vitamins and minerals, like all essential nutrients, may be beneficial or detrimental depending on the dose. For each essential nutrient, a range of intake corresponds to beneficial effects of that nutrient in both mother and baby. When intakes are below that level, the mother's health and that of the fetus falters. Health, growth, and development of the fetus are impaired when intakes of vitamins and minerals exceed beneficial levels. For some vitamins and minerals, such as vitamin A, vitamin D, iron, and selenium, the range of optimal intake is relatively narrow. For others, such as thiamin, riboflavin, and manganese, the range of optimal intake appears to be wide. It is very difficult to consume excessive levels of vitamins or minerals from food. Overdoses of vitamins and minerals are almost entirely due to the overuse of supplements.

These concerns provide the basis for the recommendation that a multivitamin and mineral supplement not be given to *all* pregnant women. Only 30 mg of iron after the twelfth week of pregnancy is recommended for all pregnant women. The preferred approach to multivitamin and mineral supplementation during pregnancy is a very reasonable one: Supplements should be prescribed like any other medication or treatment on an "as indicated" basis.

Who Should Be Taking a Multivitamin and Mineral Supplement?

A multivitamin and mineral supplement is indicated for women who:

- consume an inadequate level of vitamins and minerals in a diet that cannot be improved with nutritional guidance
- are expecting two or more babies
- are vegan
- smoke cigarettes
- use illicit drugs

• have certain illnesses or take medications that interfere with nutrient utilization by the body (for example, blood disorders, medications for seizures).

Women with specific nutrient deficiencies and those who are at risk for deficiency should be given the individual nutrients they need. If a general need for increasing nutrient intake is identified, then a specific multivitamin and mineral formulation should be recommended. Levels of vitamins and minerals needed in these situations are often markedly lower than amounts present in many of the frequently prescribed prenatal supplements. The multivitamin and mineral supplement recommended by the American College of Obstetrics and Gynecology and the Institute of Medicine of the National Academy of Sciences contains four vitamins and four minerals in the amounts indicated in Table 6–1.

If you have been given a multivitamin and mineral supplement, check the label to see how it compares to the recommended one. If it is different than the supplement described in Table 6–1 and has not been prescribed for a specific reason, and you are eating a healthy diet, you may want to think about taking the supplement less often or even if you need it at all.

Nausea and vomiting are sometimes aggravated by multivitamin and mineral supplements. It is generally recommended that

Table 6–1 Recommended Multivitamin and Mineral Supplement for Pregnancy

Nutrient	Amount	% of RDA for Pregnancy
vitamin B_6	2 mg	91
folate	300 μg	75
vitamin C	50 mg	71
vitamin D	6 μg (200 IU)	50
iron	30 mg	100
zinc	15 mg	100
copper	2 mg	100
calcium	250 mg	21

Recommended formulation is from a report on "Nutrition During Pregnancy" by the Institute of Medicine, National Academy of Sciences, 1990.

they not be taken if they make nausea and vomiting worse. Because supplement pills may look like candy to curious toddlers, partially filled bottles should not be left in a place where they can be sampled by children.

Individual Vitamin and Mineral Supplements

Individual vitamin and mineral supplements, such as vitamin C, vitamin B_6, vitamin A, or zinc should only be taken if medically indicated. Because too few studies have been done on the use of individual vitamins and minerals in pregnancy, the safety of high amounts of supplements cannot be confirmed. Very high doses of vitamins C, A, D, and B_6; and of niacin, selenium, zinc, and iodine are known to impair health in people who are not pregnant.

Individual vitamin or mineral supplements are sometimes recommended for the relief of certain problems of pregnancy, such as nausea and vomiting, preeclampsia, and preterm labor. These topics are addressed in Chapter 9.

Iron Supplements

In the United States, it is currently recommended that all pregnant women take 30 mg of iron after the twelfth week of pregnancy. This is because many women conceive with low iron stores and the supplement is needed to cover the high need for iron in pregnancy. Since iron supplements may aggravate nausea and vomiting, they should not be taken until nausea and vomiting subside; this usually happens before the twelfth week of pregnancy.

Recently, health care providers have been questioning the recommendation that all women receive an iron supplement. There is concern that too much iron is being given to women who begin pregnancy with a good level of iron stores and continue to consume sufficient amounts of iron. These women in particular may develop heartburn, cramps, and either diarrhea or constipation from excessive levels of iron. When women who do not need supplemental iron take iron pills, they do not absorb a high proportion of it. This leaves a good deal of free iron in the gut, which causes problems. Women who need iron are less likely to experience side effects from iron supplementation.

If you are experiencing side effects from iron supplements, you may want to check the dose. If it is over 30 mg per day, that may be the reason. Or you may be experiencing side effects because you don't need iron supplements. If you need the iron but are having adverse side effects from it, taking the iron supplement at bedtime, between meals, or with a glass of orange or grapefruit juice works better than taking it in a multivitamin and mineral supplement or with food.

A higher dose of iron is recommended for women who develop iron deficiency anemia in pregnancy. This subject is covered in Chapter 9.

Are Herbal Supplements Safe?

Herbal remedies are becoming a popular alternative to traditional medical therapies for some conditions that develop in pregnancy. No doubt some of the herbal remedies used are safe and effective, but there is no way to know for sure. There are no reports in the scientific literature on the safety or effectiveness of herbal remedies for pregnant women. That makes it impossible to recommend any of them.

Based on studies with nonpregnant individuals, it is clear that some herbs may cause problems. Herbs such as tonka beans, melilot, and sweet woodruff contain natural coumarins which thin the blood and may lead to delayed blood clotting. Chamomile, mandrake, pennyroyal oil, sassafras, snakeroot, and Devil's clawroot can also have quite powerful effects on the body and should be avoided during pregnancy.

Questions About Vitamin and Mineral Supplements in Pregnancy

Q. *What vitamins should I take?*

A. A vitamin supplement is not routinely recommended for pregnancy. You should take one only when necessary (see the previous section, "Who Should Be Taking a Multivitamin and Mineral

Supplement"). If a multivitamin and mineral supplement is necessary, the formulation shown in Table 6–1 is recommended. If that supplement is not available, take another one that comes close, or if you need to, take the one you have been given every other day or at an interval that would bring your daily intake in line with that advised. In rare instances, other vitamin or mineral supplements will be prescribed to meet a particular medically indicated need.

Q. *Do I have to take the supplements I was given?*

A. It depends on the reason you were given the supplement. If it was given to treat or prevent a specific problem, then yes. If it was given to you and every other pregnant woman seen without a particular reason, then maybe not. Many health care providers dispense supplements to all pregnant women because it's traditional to do so or because they think patients expect it. If you are unsure whether or not you need to take the supplement provided, ask your health care practitioner if there is a specific reason you need it.

Q. *Are calcium supplements a good substitute for milk?*

A. Milk is better than a calcium supplement. If you need to take calcium pills, make sure you are also getting vitamin D from the sun (one to two hours of sun exposure on your arms, hands, and legs per week), consuming fortified cereal or soy milk, or are taking a 200 IU vitamin D supplement daily along with the calcium. Vitamin D intake from supplements or foods should be kept between 200 and 400 IU per day. You need the vitamin D to utilize the calcium.

Q. *I find pills hard to swallow. Can you get supplements in liquid form?*

A. There may be a liquid form of the vitamin and mineral supplement recommended or prescribed. Ask your health care provider if there is one. You can crush up most supplements and swallow the pieces or mix them with food or juice. Inform your health care provider if you have problems with swallowing. Many people, however, swallow just fine but have trouble getting down large pills.

⪧ 7 ⪦

Gaining the
Right Amount of Weight

Am I having a baby or a little elephant?

—Pregnant woman's remark

P regnancy has many wonderful moments, but stepping on a scale during prenatal visits usually isn't one of them. Even though pregnant women are *supposed* to gain weight, cultural biases against weight gain often extend to pregnant women. Concerns about gaining weight can lead health care providers and women to unduly restrict it. Weight is such a loaded subject in our culture that the progress of weight gain is usually closely monitored and managed in pregnancy. But this is not the case in cultures where less importance is placed on women's weight. Without the preoccupation of maintaining a thin appearance, women are free to follow the body's hunger and fullness cues. In this situation, and food is available, women tend to gain an average of 32 pounds in pregnancy. Weight gain during pregnancy in such cultures is usually not intensely scrutinized because women do fine on their own. However, this approach doesn't work as well for many women in highly weight-conscious societies such as ours because food intake may be driven by factors other than the body's hunger and fullness signals.

If inborn systems for regulating food intake have been overridden by other motivations for eating or not eating, then it may be necessary to pay close attention to the progress of weight gain in pregnancy. The potential benefits to fetal development and growth, and the baby's future health, make it worthwhile to make sure the right amount of weight is gained during pregnancy.

The Right Amount of Weight to Gain During Pregnancy

In 1990 a scientific advisory group of the Institute of Medicine, National Academy of Sciences, released recommendations on pregnancy weight gain. Although similar reports have been issued in the past, these were the first recommendations based primarily on weight gains associated with optimal birth-weight infants. Birth weight is a primary indicator of infant health and is strongly influenced by weight gain during pregnancy. Because the amount of weight gain associated with optimal birth-weight infants varies according to the mother's weight prior to pregnancy, separate

Table 7-1 Identifying Prepregnancy Weight Status

Height		Weight Status Category		
(no shoes)	Underweight	Normal	Overweight	Obese
feet inches	*Weight in pounds (light indoor clothing)*			
4 9	92 or less	93–113	114–134	135 or more
4 10	94 or less	95–117	118–138	139 or more
4 11	97 or less	98–120	121–142	143 or more
5 0	100 or less	101–123	124–146	147 or more
5 1	103 or less	104–127	128–150	151 or more
5 2	106 or less	107–131	132–155	156 or more
5 3	109 or less	110–134	135–159	160 or more
5 4	113 or less	114–140	141–165	166 or more
5 5	117 or less	118–144	145–170	171 or more
5 6	121 or less	122–149	150–176	177 or more
5 7	124 or less	125–153	154–181	182 or more
5 8	128 or less	129–157	158–186	187 or more
5 9	131 or less	132–162	163–191	192 or more
5 10	135 or less	136–166	167–196	197 or more
5 11	139 or less	140–171	172–202	203 or more
6 0	142 or less	143–175	176–207	208 or more

Technical notes: Weight for height ranges are calculated from the 1959 Metropolitan Height and Weight Tables for Women over the age of twenty-five years. A midpoint value was determined from the range of weight and height for women of "medium frame." The cut-off point for underweight women is designated as a weight for height that is no more than 10 percent below the midpoint. The normal weight range is calculated as plus or minus 10 percent of the midpoint for each height. The overweight range is calculated as greater than 10 through 30 percent above the midpoint of weight for height. The cut-off point in weight for the obese category is calculated as a weight for height that is more than 30 percent above the midpoint of weight for height.

recommendations were made for women who enter pregnancy underweight, normal weight, overweight, or obese. Table 7–1 presents weights for height that correspond to these different prepregnancy weight status groups.

In addition, a separate recommendation was made for women pregnant with twins. Gaining the recommended amount of weight does not guarantee the delivery of healthy infants of a particular size, but it does improve the chances of a good outcome. Women who gain the suggested amounts of weight are more likely to deliver infants with robust health who feed and sleep well and who do not require special health care interventions after birth. Infants born to women who gain little weight are more likely to be preterm (born before thirty-seven weeks of gestation), small, and to require special care after delivery.

Recommended ranges of total weight gain for pregnancy are shown in Table 7–2.

Teens, women who weigh at the low end of their prepregnancy weight groups, and women who smoke are encouraged to gain weight at the higher end of the range. Women whose weights for height were at the high end of the prepregnancy weight group should gain at the lower end of the ranges. Weight gains should result from the consumption of a healthy diet.

Pattern of Weight Gain

The total pregnancy weight gains shown in Figure 7–1 should be achieved by a constant and gradual gain in weight during pregnancy. Although the pattern of weight gain normally varies somewhat, it is best if weight is not lost during any part of pregnancy.

Figure 7–1 shows the expected pattern of weight gain for women of different prepregnancy weight categories and for women expecting twins. Women generally don't gain any weight until four to six weeks after the last menstrual period, or *LMP* as abbreviated in Figure 7–1.

Rates of weight gain shown on the graph represent the middle of the recommended weight-gain ranges. Because ranges of total weight gain are recommended, and because women tend to gain weight in

Table 7–2 Recommended Weight Gain in Pregnancy

Prepregnancy	Recommended
Weight Status	Range of Weight Gain (in pounds)
A. Twin pregnancy	35–45
B. Underweight	28–40
C. Normal weight	25–35
D. Overweight	15–25
E. Obese	15

spurts rather than smoothly, weight gains that are within several pounds of those indicated on the graph are considered normal.

If you use the pregnancy weight-gain graph to chart your weight-gain progress, you should weigh yourself at approximately the same time of day while nude or wearing a similar type of clothing. Body weight normally fluctuates throughout the day, and you can get a more accurate measure of your weight gain this way.

Where Does the Weight Gain Go?

Figure 7–2 shows the approximate distribution of weight in women who gain roughly 33 pounds during pregnancy.

Only about one-third to one-fourth of a woman's total weight gain in pregnancy is represented by the fetus. The rest goes for the formation of the tissues that support fetal development and growth.

Pregnancy is accompanied by major changes in a woman's body. A major increase in blood supply, growth of the uterus and breasts, and increased fat stores support the development and growth of the fetus. The bulk of these changes begin early in pregnancy while the fetus is still very small. The body becomes prepared in the first half of pregnancy to meet the exceptionally high energy and nutrient needs of the fetus that occur during the second half of pregnancy.

Weight Gains That Go Off Track

Weight changes experienced in pregnancy may vary substantially from those recommended. There are several primary reasons why this happens. One is the intentional control of weight gain to keep

Figure 7–1 Pregnancy Weight Gain Graph

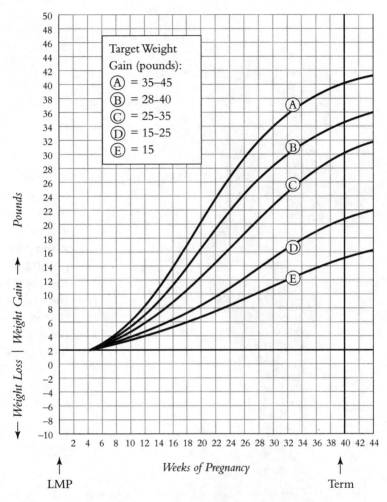

Source: Reprinted with permission of Judith E. Brown © 1997.

it low. Restriction of weight gain early and late in pregnancy is particularly common among women who enter pregnancy overweight and those who are very concerned about their weight.

Nausea and vomiting is a second reason why weight gain may go awry. Women with nausea and vomiting in early pregnancy may find it hard to gain weight. Although it used to be thought that weight loss early in pregnancy due to nausea and vomiting was

Figure 7–2 Where Does All the Weight Go?

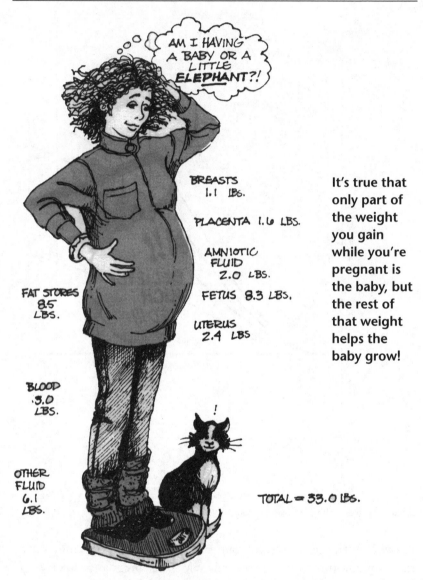

Here's where the weight goes for a woman who gains 33 pounds.

Source: This illustration was developed for an educational program on nutrition and pregnancy sponsored by the Maternal and Child Health Bureau of the Public Health Service.

okay if the weight was gained back later, it now appears that the best situation is a continuous, gradual weight gain. For women with nausea and vomiting, it may be necessary to snack, to separate the ingestion of liquid and solid foods, and to eat foods that are well tolerated. (Specific advice for diet during nausea and vomiting is given in Chapter 9.)

A third reason for weight gains that do not follow the graph is water retention. Some women accumulate large amounts of water in addition to that needed for blood volume expansion and other purposes. An increased body content of water may be reflected in an unexpected weight gain. A high level of water accumulation can sometimes be identified by edema, or the swelling of the hands, ankles, and feet. Unless accompanied by elevated blood pressure and protein in the urine, such an accumulation of water is considered normal. In fact, women who experience edema without hypertension or protein in the urine are more likely to have healthy-sized infants than are women who do not do so. The extra water that accumulates will be lost within a few days after delivery. If weight gain is due to water retention and not to an excessive intake of calories or a major reduction in physical activity level, there is no need to cut back on your food intake. Women who unexpectedly gain weight rapidly, such as two to four pounds in a week after twenty or so weeks of pregnancy, may be developing a condition called preeclampsia. Consequently, any unexpected rapid gain in weight should be brought to the attention of your health care provider.

Preeclampsia occurs in about 7 percent of first pregnancies and is often signaled by a rapid weight gain, protein spillage into the urine, abnormally high blood pressure, and sometimes edema. This condition is unique to pregnancy and may be mild or severe, depending on the elevation in blood pressure. Other symptoms of preeclampsia include visual disturbances, headache, elevated hemoglobin level, and stomach pain.

Weight gain may go off-track if women consume too much food. Women who substantially lower their levels of physical activity due to bed rest, an injury, or other reason may gain more weight than expected if food intake doesn't change. If the rate of weight gain becomes too high, smaller meals and snacks are indicated.

Periods of excessively high weight gain during pregnancy should not be offset with weight loss. Rather, it is recommended that women slow down their rate of weight gain by eating less or exercising more. Weight loss in pregnancy is never recommended! Weight-loss programs should not be started until after delivery, and not be so severe as to compromise the level of breast milk production in women who breast-feed. (Read more about this topic in Chapter 12.)

Weight Loss After Pregnancy

If the success of weight-loss programs is measured by the amount of weight lost, then delivery is a highly successful weight-loss program! Women generally lose 15 pounds within a few days after delivery and approximately 24 pounds by six to eight weeks postpartum. Breast-feeding increases weight loss somewhat in most women, although breast-feeding women are encouraged not to lose weight too quickly because it may compromise breast milk supply. On average, women who gain within the recommended ranges weigh about 2 pounds more twelve months after delivery than they did prior to pregnancy. Women who gain below the recommended ranges tend to weigh approximately 1 to 2 pounds more twelve months after delivery than they did before pregnancy. Body weights tend to be 5 or more pounds higher a year after delivery among women who gain above the recommended ranges.

Weight retention after pregnancy varies a good deal among individual women. Some women begin to gain weight after delivery due to changes in eating habits or physical activity levels. Other women lose weight rather quickly. It is hard to predict how much weight an individual woman will lose after delivery. It is clear, however, that women who gain weight excessively will have more to lose after their babies are born. A reasonable rate of weight loss in the weeks that follow delivery is 1 to 2 pounds per week. Losing weight faster may drain your energy level, make you more susceptible to illness, and reduce breast milk volume. Be kind to yourself and don't try to lose weight too rapidly after pregnancy. With a new baby around, you will need all the energy and stamina you can muster.

Questions About Weight Gain and Pregnancy

Q. *How much should my baby weigh at birth?*

A. Optimal birth weights based on the lowest risk of death and health problems are between 3,500 and 4,500 grams (7 pounds, 12 ounces to 9 pounds, 14 ounces). Some babies, however, are naturally smaller or larger than others and are of robust health. The chances of being optimally healthy at birth, however, are higher for infants who weigh within the optimal range. Recommended weight-gain goals are based on the delivery of infants with optimal birth weight. That doesn't always happen, though, because other factors such as smoking during pregnancy, preterm delivery, the size of the mother, and the development of hypertension or diabetes in pregnancy, as well as other conditions, also affect birth weight.

Q. *Should African American women gain a different amount of weight than Caucasian women?*

A. No, the recommendations are the same. Neither race nor ethnicity should be a factor in advice given about weight gain during pregnancy.

Q. *How much weight should I gain?*

A. Just like panty hose, no one size fits all. How much weight you should gain in pregnancy primarily depends on your weight before conception and whether you are expecting two or more infants. Table 7–2 shows the recommended weight gains for pregnancy.

Q. *Will the amount of weight I gain affect the chances that I'll deliver early?*

A. Weight gain in the second half of pregnancy is related to the risk of preterm delivery. Underweight and normal-weight women who gain less than 0.8 pounds per week, and overweight and obese women gaining less than 0.7 pounds per week in the third trimester, have a higher risk of delivering early. Low rates of weight gain in the first half of pregnancy are more closely related to the birth of small infants, especially among women who begin pregnancy underweight.

Q. *How do I know I'm gaining the right amount of weight?*

A. First identify your prepregnancy weight status group (Table 7–1). Then plot your weight gain on the graph in Figure 7–1. As long as you are consistently gaining some weight, don't worry if your weight differs from that shown on the graph by a few pounds.

Q. *Why should I gain 30 pounds if the baby will only weigh around 8 pounds at birth?*

A. You can't build a car unless you have a factory.

Most of the weight gained in pregnancy goes into the development of tissues that allow fetal development, growth, and breast-feeding. Women must build up a variety of tissues that will support the nourishment of the fetus. These tissues are responsible for the bulk of weight gain during pregnancy. If weight gain is too low, these tissues are not fully developed nor functional and fetal development and growth may be compromised.

Q. *If I started pregnancy overweight, is it okay to lose weight during pregnancy?*

A. No, it is never considered wise to lose weight during pregnancy. Women who begin pregnancy with extra fat stores do not need to gain as much weight as women who have less stored fat. Some of the energy required by the fetus can be obtained from fat stores brought into pregnancy. However, because the fetus needs a constant supply of glucose, it is best to consume enough food to gain weight at a low and gradual pace from four weeks of pregnancy onward.

Q. *I started pregnancy overweight and have been careful to eat a healthy diet since I found out I was pregnant. The thing is, I've been losing weight ever since I started to eat healthy. Does it matter if I lose weight if I'm eating a really good diet?*

A. You should gain some weight. Eat more healthy foods.

It is fairly common for women who are overweight to lose weight if they change to a more nutrient-dense diet during pregnancy. Although it is excellent that your food choices are healthy ones, you still need to gain weight. The fetus is more adversely affected by weight loss or fasting during pregnancy than is the mother. Weight loss in pregnancy may mean the fetus is using too much fat for energy and not enough glucose. It may also reduce the increase in maternal blood volume and compromise the delivery of nutrients and other substances needed by the fetus.

Q. *I'm gaining too much weight. How can I cut down?*

A. Weight gain during pregnancy may occur in spurts of several pounds within a few days or a week. If this occurs because you have been very hungry and have eaten in response to this, don't worry much about short-term weight gain. Your appetite will probably decrease with time. If you are gaining too much weight and have not eaten that much, you may be retaining fluid. If weight gain is due to water, you shouldn't cut back on your food intake. Tell your health care provider that you are gaining more weight than you expect given the amount of food you are eating and the exercise you are getting. Your health care provider may want to check to make sure your blood pressure is okay.

If your weight-gain pattern over several weeks to a month is too high because you are eating too much, then it's time to reduce portion sizes and perhaps to eat fewer snacks. Foods that contribute the least nutritional value should be the first ones deleted from your diet. Increasing physical activity can also help slow your rate of gain. But remember, keep your pattern of weight gain positive.

Q. *How much weight gain is too much?*

A. If you enter pregnancy underweight, about 45 pounds; if normal weight, 42 to 44 pounds; if overweight, 34 pounds; and if obese, gaining more than about 20 pounds is considered excessive. The primary problem associated with substantial weight gain in pregnancy is having to lose the excess weight after delivery.

Q. *If I gain the recommended amount of weight, how much weight will I have to lose after my baby is born?*

A. On average, women will have about 2 extra pounds to lose if they gain the recommended amount of weight. Women who gain more than the recommended amount will have more weight to lose, and women who gain less tend to have only 1 pound to lose. Weight should be lost gradually. Weight gain occurred across nine months of pregnancy and there is no reason to expect it all will be lost within a few weeks or months after delivery.

Q. *What problems are caused by gaining too much weight during pregnancy?*

A. There are several possibilities:
1. You'll have more weight to lose after delivery.
2. You may have a baby that is large and must be delivered by cesarean section (although this is an uncommon reason for a C-section).
3. You may be unhappy about your weight gain.

Large weight gains in healthy pregnant women are actually associated with very few complications. The biggest concern for normal weight and underweight women is weight retention after delivery.

Q. *My partner is tall. Does that mean the baby will be big?*

A. The father's size is not related to birth weight. However, it is related to the eventual height of children.

Q. *My partner has gained more weight than I have this pregnancy. What can I do to help?*

A. Aha! A sympathetic pregnancy!

It isn't all that uncommon for partners to gain weight during pregnancy; the gain may be related to the presence of more food in the household and more eating opportunities. Perhaps your partner can plan reductions in the amount of food that will be eaten at meals and snacks. That would be a good start. Your partner should also not gauge how much is eaten based on when and how much you eat.

⮜ 8 ⮞

Recommendations for Exercise in Pregnancy

Reading is to the mind what exercise is to the body.

—Sir Richard Steele, 1712

Regular exercise is something many women do not want to give up and that other women want to take up during pregnancy. Unfortunately, deciding what to do about prenatal exercise can be troublesome. Women who seek out opinions on the safety and benefits of regular exercise in pregnancy hear both enthusiastic reports of its benefits and stern warnings about its dire consequences. What is the scoop on exercise in pregnancy? Is it safe and beneficial for mother and baby, or might it be hazardous? This chapter addresses the current status of knowledge about and recommendations for exercise in pregnancy, and answers questions women frequently ask about this topic.

Overview of Exercise in Pregnancy

About 42 percent of pregnant women in the United States exercise, and most of these women walk, swim, or participate in other aerobic exercises. In general, women avoid heavy physical activity and reduce their levels of exercise as pregnancy progresses. Prepregnancy physical activity routines are often modified due to changes in balance, the increase in blood volume (which can cause women to tire more easily), the presence of nausea and vomiting and other discomforts, and weight gain. Levels of physical activity generally rise again after delivery when there is a new baby to care for and a drive to get back into shape. Activities that "feel right" often include:

- walking
- swimming
- stretching
- golf
- Frisbee
- tennis
- floor exercises (aerobics, stretching, and front- and side-standing leg lifts).

Effects of Exercise During Pregnancy

Both the potential benefits and hazards of exercise in pregnancy have been overstated in the past. Current evidence indicates that regular physical activity in healthy, well-nourished women is safe and may be somewhat beneficial. Women who exercise moderately and regularly tend to experience fewer of the normal discomforts of pregnancy and benefit from the sense of well-being regular exercise can bring. Women who consume a healthy diet, gain weight at the recommended level, and avoid activities that are too intense or may cause injury should not worry that exercise will harm their baby.

There are some women for whom exercise during pregnancy is a matter for concern. Exercise may not be advised for women who fail to gain weight, or who have preeclampsia, premature rupture of the membrane, hypertension, heart disease, preterm labor, second or third trimester bleeding, or a weak cervix. Pregnant women should also be sure to exercise moderately, and not "overdo it."

The Upper Limits of Exercise During Pregnancy

Excessive levels of physical activity in pregnancy can reduce fetal growth and increase the risk of preterm delivery. A cardinal sign that exercise level is too high is a low rate of weight gain. Exercise or physical activity that ends in exhaustion, endurance activities, and activities undertaken in hot, humid climates should be out-of-bounds for pregnant women.

Recommendations for Exercise in Pregnancy

The American College of Obstetrics and Gynecology and other groups have studied the benefits and hazards of physical activity in pregnancy and developed recommendations for exercise. These recommendations are highlighted in Table 8–1.

Current recommendations for exercise in pregnancy are less restrictive than in the past and reflect the conclusion that moderate levels of physical activity by healthy, well-nourished women pose no special risk to pregnancy. Pregnant women should exercise moderately, or at 50 to 60 percent of maximal heart rate for twenty to thirty minutes three times per week. Maximal heart rate, or MHR, represents your maximal oxygen utilization level, or VO_2 max. Maximal heart rate represents the highest number of times your heart can beat per minute during periods of highly intense

Table 8–1 Recommendations for Exercise in Pregnancy

The Dos
- Do exercise moderately and regularly unless otherwise advised by your health care provider.
- Do emphasize non–weight bearing activities and those that don't require a keen sense of balance.
- Do wear loose-fitting, lightweight clothing that allows heat to escape and moisture to evaporate.
- Do drink plenty of fluids during exercise; eat appropriately.
- Do consume a healthy diet and gain weight as recommended.
- Do exercise at 50 to 60 percent of maximal heart rate (or VO_2 max).

The Don'ts
- Don't exercise or perform physical work to exhaustion. Quit when you feel tired.
- Don't exercise while laying on your back in the second and third trimester.
- Don't exercise in hot, humid conditions.
- Don't perform activities that may traumatize the abdomen or uterus or cause you to lose your balance.
- Don't fast or exercise while you are hungry.

exercise. Brief bouts of exercise at 70 percent of MHR are considered okay. You can estimate your MHR from your age: 100 percent of MHR is estimated as 220 minus a person's age. (This formula may be somewhat undependable for pregnant women, who tend to have a higher heart rate than nonpregnant women.) To calculate 50 percent of MHR for a thirty-one-year-old, for example, you would subtract 30 from 220 and multiply the results times 0.5:

$$220 - 30 = 190$$
$$190 \times 0.5 = 95 \text{ beats per minute}$$

Exercise that results in a heart rate of 95 beats per minute would approximately equal 50 percent of MHR. To see if you are exercising at this level, you need to take your pulse and determine how many times your heart beats within a minute. Usually people count the number of pulses in ten seconds and then multiply that figure times 6 to calculate beats per minute.

Specific concerns about what exercises or levels of physical activity are safe and questions about how the presence of certain physical problems relate to exercise in pregnancy should be brought to the attention of your health care provider.

Questions About Exercise and Pregnancy

Q. *Can I alter my physical activity level to help manage my weight gain?*

A. Yes. Increasing low levels, or decreasing high levels of physical activity helps some women achieve the recommended weight-gain goals. Intense exercise should not be used, however, to lose weight. Weight loss is never recommended in pregnancy.

Q. *Are high levels of physical activity harmful to the baby?*

A. They can be harmful if too much of the mother's energy supply is going to fuel exercise and too little is available for the fetus. Blood glucose levels drop more quickly with exercise when women are pregnant because of fetal demands for glucose. Blood and oxygen supply to the fetus may be compromised when women exercise strenuously or undertake endurance events. Exercise in hot, humid climates may lead to overheating and dehydration, both of which can be harmful to both mother and baby.

Q. *If I exercise during pregnancy will my labor be shorter?*

A. There is no clear answer to this question. Although it does not appear that exercise during pregnancy is related to longer labors, it is not clear that it decreases the length of labor.

Q. *Is there any harm in not exercising during pregnancy?*

A. Women who don't exercise during pregnancy may experience more of the aches and pains that can accompany pregnancy and may tire more easily than women who exercise regularly. Otherwise, few differences in physical health have been observed between active and sedentary pregnant women.

Q. *Are there particular exercises I should avoid during pregnancy?*

A. Highly strenuous exercises, those that require a keen sense of balance, and exercises that may traumatize the uterus or abdomen should not be undertaken. This eliminates endurance events, hauling heavy objects, water skiing, scuba diving, surfing, inline skating, ice skating, downhill skiing, horseback riding, sit-ups, push-ups, toe-touches, and field hockey and other contact sports.

Q. *Exercises I used to do all the time are more difficult now that I'm pregnant. Is that normal?*

A. Yes, it's normal. Many women tire more easily from physical activity, especially during the first few months of pregnancy. Added blood volume, more weight, and shifting balance all contribute to making exercise harder when pregnant.

If you tire very easily or feel fatigued most of the time even though you are getting a good night's sleep, make sure you don't have anemia. Have your health care provider check for it.

Nutritional Aids
for Common Problems
in Pregnancy

*"This pregnancy has been full of surprises," quipped
Crystal to her friend, who was also pregnant. "I was
expecting a baby and not morning sickness, heartburn,
and leg cramps that strike like a bolt of lightning in the
middle of the night!"*

*"So you're going through that, too," Crystal's friend
replied thoughtfully. "I wish I had known that sooner.
It would have taken a lot of the worry out of these
pregnancy surprises."*

I t is rare that women complete pregnancy without experiencing
nausea, vomiting, leg cramps, constipation, heartburn, backaches,
or other common side effects. It is also rare that they aren't taken
by surprise by their occurrence. The purpose of this chapter is to
help you avoid these surprises and to present ways you can help
relieve the discomfort they can cause.

This chapter examines six conditions of pregnancy that may be
managed through nutrition:
• nausea and vomiting
• constipation
• heartburn
• iron deficiency anemia
• gestational diabetes
• preeclampsia

Because each of these conditions can become severe or may signal other problems, they should be monitored by your health care provider and treated medically as needed.

Nausea and Vomiting

Why nausea, or nausea with vomiting, occurs during most pregnancies is one of the great mysteries of obstetrics. The presence of these symptoms appears to be related to hormonal changes and generally indicate that pregnancy is progressing well. Well, that is, for the fetus. The mother, on the other hand, may be miserable. Nausea or nausea and vomiting tend to start around two to four weeks after conception and decline gradually or abruptly end some time during the third month. For 10 to 30 percent of women, nausea or nausea and vomiting last throughout pregnancy and are only cured by delivery. Although often referred to as "morning sickness," nausea and vomiting are not confined to the morning hours in most cases.

Nausea and vomiting that are regular, hard to stop, and that causes weight loss and dehydration (signaled by fatigue, a low urine output, and dark yellow urine) is referred to as *hyperemesis gravidarum,* or *hyperemesis,* for short. Women with this form of severe nausea and vomiting require close medical supervision. The goal of medical care for hyperemesis is to stop the nausea and vomiting, to remedy dehydration, and to enable women to resume food intake and weight gain. There is a light at the end of this tunnel, however. Women with hyperemesis or less severe cases of nausea and vomiting who stay well hydrated, eat a healthy diet, and gain weight appropriately frequently deliver very healthy infants.

Nausea and Vomiting Triggers

Women with nausea and vomiting or hyperemesis are often highly sensitive to certain odors and become queasy if they smell the wrong aromas. (Just reading about the association between odors and nausea may be enough to push some women's "queasy" buttons. If that's you, skip over the rest of this paragraph.) Odors known to trigger nausea and vomiting in some women include that of fresh and old coffee, vitamin supplements, cleaning agents, perfume, aerosol room fresheners, cigarette and cigar smoke, dirty diapers, garbage, and gas and diesel fumes. Clean, cool air in an odorless environment is generally found to be soothing.

Iron supplements aggravate nausea and vomiting in many women and are not recommended for the first trimester of pregnancy. Generally, their use should be discontinued until women are feeling better if they contribute to nausea and vomiting later in pregnancy.

Prevention and Treatment of Nausea and Vomiting

It is not known how to prevent nausea and vomiting from occurring, but there are actions women can take that may help reduce the frequency and severity of both:

1. Snack on dry foods often.

Nausea and vomiting are more likely to occur on an empty stomach, so frequent snacks may help. Dry, high-carbohydrate foods, such as crackers, vanilla wafers, dry toast, or dry cereals often go down easily and stay down. Snacking on such foods before you get out of bed in the morning may help prevent a queasy morning stomach. A wide variety of other foods have been found to help prevent nausea and vomiting. Because the best choices are different for individual women, you will be the best judge of what foods are most easily tolerated. If potato chips, hard-boiled eggs, yogurt, or canned fruits sound good to you, for example, try them. It is better to eat the foods you can keep down than to not eat enough to gain some weight.

2. Separate your intake of solids and liquids.

Eating small meals or snacks about every two hours while you are awake and drinking fluids about half an hour after solid foods may help prevent nausea and vomiting. Some beverages are better at settling the stomach than others. For some women, warm milk with a bit of sugar or pasteurized honey tastes good, while lemonade, iced tea, water, fruit juices, V-8 juice, tomato juice, sports drinks, ginger ale, or fruit-flavored sodas work for other women. Sometimes room-temperature beverages or "flat" sodas are easily tolerated. Ice chips or very cold beverages are preferred by some women because they help foods stay down. Because the need for water increases during bouts of vomiting, women with vomiting should drink ample amounts of beverages that are well tolerated.

3. Stay away from odors or tastes that make you queasy.

Following this recommendation may take advance planning and some help. You may need to buy prepackaged meals or have someone else do the cooking, buy gasoline at the full-service aisle (so you can avoid smelling the fumes), or give up foods that make you feel nauseous.

4. Consider some other factors.

Some women find that nausea and vomiting are set off by brushing their teeth shortly after they wake up. Carefully brushing your teeth later can help prevent this.

Since iron supplements may aggravate nausea and vomiting, it is recommended that their use be discontinued, at least temporarily, if nausea and vomiting are a problem.

Medications for Nausea and Vomiting

Nausea and vomiting persist in some women despite their best efforts to control it. For these women, medications such as pyridoxine (vitamin B$_6$), doxylamine, and special high-carbohydrate solutions may be given under the supervision of the health care provider. Hospitalization may be required in severe cases of nausea and vomiting.

Other Causes of Nausea and Vomiting

Nausea and vomiting can be due to causes other than pregnancy. Because it may signal other health problems, it is always a good idea to get the reason for nausea and vomiting diagnosed by your health care provider.

Constipation

Constipation is characterized by abdominal pain, difficult and infrequent bowel movements, and the passage of hard stools. Worry, anxiety, a low level of exercise, and a low-fiber diet are common causes of constipation. In rare instances, constipation is related to intestinal blockages, the excessive use of laxatives, or the use of medications that cause constipation as a side effect. Constipation in pregnancy is thought to be due to hormones that relax the intestinal muscles and to the pressure caused by the expanding uterus on the intestines. It can occur anytime, but is most common late in pregnancy.

Prevention and Treatment of Constipation

There are several approaches to the prevention and treatment of constipation:

1. Eat a high-fiber diet.

Consumption of 25 to 30 g per day of dietary fiber from fruits and vegetables, high-fiber breakfast cereals, bran, and powdered bulk-forming supplemental fiber such as psyllium or methyl cellulose can help prevent and relieve constipation. Table 2–2 lists food sources of fiber. It is best to check out the fiber value of foods rather than make assumptions about which ones are high in fiber. Not all foods thought of as being high in fiber actually are. Because greater consumption of fiber increases your requirement for water, you'll need to make sure you drink more fluids. You know you are consuming enough fiber and fluid when your stools are large and soft. Too much fiber can lead to diarrhea.

Prunes, prune juice, and figs also help relieve constipation. Although they are not particularly high in fiber, prunes and figs contain other substances that speed up elimination.

2. Drink 10 to 12 cups of fluid each day.

The combination of fiber and fluids is what enhances elimination, and both are necessary. Women who sweat a lot or are exposed to hot, humid climates may need more than 10 to 12 cups of fluid each day.

3. Exercise.

Inactivity fosters constipation. Walking, swimming, or other moderate exercise helps mobilize the intestines.

4. Cut back on iron supplements.

Iron supplements cause constipation in some women, especially if the dose is high (over 30 mg per day). Constipation will often improve if the amount of supplemental iron taken is reduced or if smaller doses of iron are taken at one time. Women with good iron levels and a healthy diet do not need to take iron supplements at all.

Laxative pills are not recommended for the treatment of constipation during pregnancy because they may stimulate uterine contractions. Mineral oil is not advised, either, because it substantially reduces nutrient absorption.

Heartburn

Heartburn, or "acid indigestion" occurs when acidic fluids in the stomach spurt up into the esophagus. Although stomach juices should only go down the digestive tract, they can back up if pressure on the stomach is high or if the valve that closes the top of the stomach becomes relaxed. Both of these factors seem to play a role in the development of heartburn during pregnancy. Between 30 and 50 percent of women experience heartburn, especially late in pregnancy when the fetus exerts strong, upward pressure on the stomach. Heartburn can, however, occur during any part of pregnancy.

Prevention and Treatment of Heartburn

The symptoms of heartburn can often be alleviated by one or more of the following measures:

1. Consume small meals and snacks.

Pressure on the stomach is higher when it is full.

2. Don't eat a meal within three hours of bedtime.

Lying down with a full stomach increases the likelihood that acidic stomach fluids will escape into the esophagus. The stomach usually empties about three hours after a meal.

3. Reduce the use of iron supplements.

If iron supplements give you heartburn, the dose of iron is probably too high. If iron is needed, take a lower dose at bedtime with orange or grapefruit juice.

4. Position your body in ways that reduce heartburn.

Bending over may worsen heartburn, so try to avoid doing so. Sleeping with your head elevated may also help reduce heartburn.

5. In some cases, use medications for heartburn.

Antacids such as Tums that act in the stomach rather than pills for heartburn may be advised by your health care provider.

Iron Deficiency Anemia

Iron deficiency anemia is fairly common in pregnancy and is related to preterm delivery and the birth of small infants. In women, iron deficiency generally reduces appetite, food intake, mental alertness, and productivity. It can cause irritability, fatigue, and an increased susceptibility to infection as well. Iron deficiency anemia is especially common among women who have previously experienced it, who donate blood regularly, who habitually consume a low-iron diet, who have had a previous cesarean section, and who enter pregnancy with low iron stores.

Iron deficiency anemia is usually diagnosed when blood hemoglobin levels in the first trimester are less than 11 g/dl, less than 10.5 g/dl in the second trimester, or less than 11 g/dl in the third trimester. Iron deficiency anemia is also diagnosed when ferritin levels (a measure of iron stores) are less than 15 µg/ml (or sometimes less than 12 μg/ml). Hemoglobin levels between 10.5 and 13.2 g/dl in the second and third trimester of pregnancy are considered ideal. Levels of hemoglobin normally decrease in pregnancy due to an increase in blood volume. Among women without iron deficiencies, hemoglobin levels do not increase with iron supplements.

There is a tendency among U.S. health care providers to dispense doses of iron that are too high and cause side effects. Only 30 mg of iron daily in the second and third trimester of pregnancy is needed to prevent iron deficiency, and 30 to 60 mg per day to treat it. Women with good iron stores do not absorb as much iron from supplements as do women who need the iron. Unabsorbed iron in the gut can produce nausea, heartburn, gas, cramps, diarrhea, and constipation. Stools produced when too much iron is taken are generally tarry, dark, and dense.

Rather than take excessive levels of iron and put up with the side effects, about one-third of pregnant women will stop taking their iron pills. All too often, the leftover pills are put into a medicine cabinet and later found by curious toddlers. Iron overdose is the leading cause of poisoning deaths in young children in the United States. Use of excessively high amounts of iron in supplements can lead to another problem—women may not take them even if they are needed, and so may develop iron deficiency later on or in the next pregnancy. How much better it would be if the proper amount of iron was given in the first place! Overloading women with iron in pregnancy is an out-of-date practice, one that is changing too slowly.

A new school of thought about the use of iron supplements by all pregnant women is emerging in the United States and Europe. Scientists are calling for a reexamination of the recommendation that all pregnant women receive iron. Iron supplements should be prescribed based on each woman's need for iron. Women who have a good level of stored iron and who consume iron and vitamin C–rich foods probably do not need iron supplements.

Prevention and Treatment of Iron Deficiency Anemia

The use of 30 mg of iron daily in the second and third trimester is currently recommended for the prevention of iron deficiency anemia in pregnancy. For women who have iron deficiency anemia, 30 to 60 mg of iron should be taken daily. If higher doses of iron are prescribed, a 15 mg zinc supplement and a 2 mg copper supplement should be added. The reason additional zinc and copper are needed is because of the effect of high doses of supplemental iron on zinc and copper levels. Iron from supplements is better absorbed if taken in small doses with orange or grapefruit juice several times during the day.

Gestational Diabetes

Gestational diabetes occurs in 3 to 6 percent of pregnant women overall. It is defined as carbohydrate intolerance that begins in pregnancy and is characterized by high blood glucose levels. Because high blood glucose levels in pregnancy impair fetal growth and may threaten fetal survival, pregnant women in many countries are given a screening test for this condition between twenty-four and twenty-eight weeks of pregnancy. If this test is positive, a three-hour oral glucose tolerance test is given. If blood glucose levels are found to be high, the diagnosis of gestational diabetes is made.

Gestational diabetes in three out of four women can be managed by diet; one in four requires both a special diet and insulin injections. Insulin may be recommended if dietary control of blood glucose levels is not achieved within a week or two after the diagnosis of gestational diabetes. Very high blood glucose levels may be treated with insulin immediately.

The primary goal of the treatment of gestational diabetes is the delivery of a healthy baby. This is most likely to occur if blood glucose levels remain within the normal range during pregnancy.

Prevention and Treatment of Gestational Diabetes

Little is known about the prevention of gestational diabetes. Although it is difficult to predict which individuals will develop this condition, women who enter pregnancy obese, who had gestational diabetes in a previous pregnancy, or who are over the age of thirty-five develop gestational diabetes more often than other women.

The management of gestational diabetes generally involves eating a prescribed diet; monitoring food intake, blood glucose levels, and weight; exercise; and (if needed) insulin injections. Women with gestational diabetes often attend instructional classes and many health care providers organize support groups for them.

Diet is the mainstay of the treatment of gestational diabetes whether women use insulin or not. To achieve good control of blood glucose levels, diets have to be individually developed (preferably by a registered dietitian with expertise in gestational diabetes) based on a woman's blood glucose level, weight, exercise habits, and food preferences. Because protein and fat in foods raise the blood glucose levels less than carbohydrates, diets prescribed for women with gestational diabetes are relatively high in protein and fat and low in carbohydrate. The number of calories prescribed and the amount of protein, fat, and carbohydrate in the diet is often modified during the course of pregnancy depending on blood glucose control and weight gain.

Because diets for women with gestational diabetes have to be individualized and blood glucose response to the diet monitored, there is no one dietary prescription that fits all women with this problem. There are, however, several common characteristics of recommended diets:

1. Caloric intake is set at a level that promotes adequate weight gain.

The weight-gain goals for women with gestational diabetes are the same as those for women without this condition. Since both weight loss and excessive weight gain can interfere with fetal growth, development, and health and impair blood glucose control, weight gain among women with gestational diabetes should stay within the recommended range.

2. The diet provides all of the nutrients needed for pregnancy.

Diets prescribed for women with gestational diabetes contain a healthy array of foods. No special foods are required, but women should restrict their intake of sweets. Artificial sweeteners do not raise blood glucose levels and are okay to use.

3. Food intake is divided into three meals and one to three snacks.

Regular, preplanned meals and snacks are a key element in blood glucose control. Because carbohydrates in food raise blood glucose levels the most, intake of high-carbohydrate foods is spread out across the day's meals and snacks. Breakfast often contains the least carbohydrate. Women with gestational diabetes may be taught to "carbohydrate count" to help them plan their carbohydrate intake for the day.

If insulin is necessary, dietary prescriptions will be adjusted to account for the reduced blood glucose levels that result from insulin. To keep blood glucose levels normal, it is important to remain on the prescribed diet when insulin is used.

Exercise

Exercise is often recommended for women with gestational diabetes because it may improve blood glucose control. Walking, swimming, aerobic dancing, bicycling, and resistance exercises are a few of the options for the low-to-moderate-intensity activities recommended. Women are generally encouraged to spend twenty to thirty minutes three times per week exercising. Additional information about exercise in pregnancy is given in Chapter 8.

Dr. Lois Jovanovic-Peterson, an internationally known expert on gestational diabetes, offers this specific advice for working exercise into the lives of inactive women. She suggests women exercise at home while watching the news. With two large cans of tomato sauce from the cupboard, find a sturdy chair with firm back support. Lift each can above your head with one hand five times and then lift both cans together for five times. Continue this for twenty minutes or until the sports comes on the news. (Be careful not to drop the cans when you have them over your head!) If after twenty minutes you are unable to sing in one breath "row, row, row your boat gently down the stream," you have had a cardiovascular workout. If you can, increase the weight you lift as time goes on.

Preeclampsia

Preeclampsia is a condition unique to pregnancy and the first twenty-four hours after delivery. It occurs in about 7 percent of first pregnancies and is characterized by high blood pressure and protein in the urine. Edema, or swelling, often accompanies preeclampsia. The cause of preeclampsia is not known, but it is thought to reflect a kidney disorder. Although it begins to develop very early in pregnancy, preeclampsia is usually not diagnosed until the third trimester. A rapid weight gain in the second half of pregnancy, swelling, elevated hemoglobin, reduced urine output, nausea, stomach pain, headache, and impaired vision are signs of this disorder. Although it is difficult to predict who will develop preeclampsia, women having their first babies and underweight, poorly nourished, and heavy women are at a higher risk.

There is no cure for preeclampsia. However, women diagnosed with it may be put on bed rest or given medications to reduce blood pressure. Although not officially recommended, some health care providers give women with preeclampsia 1.5 to 2.0 grams of calcium per day. Calcium supplements often effectively reduce blood pressure and appear to have few side effects. Preeclampsia should not be treated by restricting weight gain, caloric intake, fluids, or salt (sodium). These interventions not only don't work, but may be harmful to both mother and fetus.

Diets high in fish, fish oils, and other oils have been reported to decrease the incidence of preeclampsia. The safety and effectiveness of this approach still is under investigation. Although several herbal, chiropractic, and other alternative remedies for preeclampsia have been proposed, their effectiveness and safety have not been scientifically demonstrated.

10

Nutrition and Twin Pregnancy: Special Considerations

An ounce of prevention is worth two pounds of cure.

If you are expecting two or more babies, eating well and gaining the right amount of weight can make an impressive difference in your health during pregnancy as well as the health of your babies. This chapter presents information that is often not covered in prenatal care but may represent the ounce of prevention that is worth well over two pounds of cure.

Dietary intake and weight gain during twin pregnancy requires special attention for several reasons. Energy and nutrient needs, and stresses on the mother's body, are high during twin pregnancy. Because twin pregnancies are generally two to three weeks shorter than singleton pregnancies, there is a need to eat right and gain weight as early in pregnancy as possible. In addition, the healthier women remain during pregnancy, the better prepared they will be for the hectic life that arrives along with twins.

This chapter highlights differences in diet and weight-gain recommendations for twin versus singleton pregnancy. For questions related to other aspects of nutrition for pregnancy, please refer to Chapters 4 through 9 covering specific topics.

Diet for Twin Pregnancy

Dietary recommendations for women expecting twins differ in only one respect from those presented earlier. Women expecting twins need higher levels of energy and nutrients in their diets.

Table 10–1 presents a food group guide for selecting a diet that provides the nutrients needed by women having twins.

Individual women may need to consume fewer servings of foods within the food groups, or more, depending on their rate of weight gain. Because of the amount of food needed by women nourishing twins, frequent snacks are in order.

Table 10–1   A Dietary Intake Guide for Twin Pregnancy

Food Guide Pyramid Group	Standard serving sizes	Suggested servings per day
1. Bread, cereal, rice, and pasta	bread, 1 slice cereal, 1 cup hot cereal, ½ cup bagel, ½ rice or pasta, ½ cup tortilla, 1	8–13
2. Vegetables	raw or cooked, ½ cup leafy, 1 cup juice, ¾ cup	4–6
3. Fruits	fresh, 1 piece canned, ½ cup juice, ¾ cup	3–5
4. Milk, yogurt, and cheese	milk, 1 cup soy milk, 1 cup yogurt, 1 cup cottage cheese, ½ cup cheese, 1½ ounces	4
5. Meat, poultry, fish, dry beans, eggs, and nuts	meat, 3 ounces dried beans, ½ cup tofu, ½ cup eggs, 2 peanut butter, 4 tablespoons	3–4
6. Fats, oils, and sweets	fats and oils, 2 teaspoons sweets, 1 ounce	As needed for weight gain

Weight Gain Recommendations for Twin Pregnancy

Women having twins need to gain more weight than other pregnant women. In addition, relatively high rates of weight gain should begin early in pregnancy. Gaining weight early in pregnancy represents a particular challenge for many women with twins because nausea and vomiting are more likely in twin pregnancy and they are often more severe. Guidance given in Chapter 9 on the nutritional management of this problem may be helpful for women who have a poor appetite due to nausea or who have a tough time keeping food down. It is best to gain weight when experiencing nausea and vomiting if at all possible. If your appetite is poor for other reasons, you may have to schedule regular eating times and eat "by the clock" rather than in response to appetite.

How much weight women pregnant with twins should gain during pregnancy depends on their prepregnant weight. Women coming into pregnancy with an ample supply of fat stores should gain approximately 25 to 35 pounds, or roughly ¾ to 1 pound per week. Women who begin pregnancy at normal weight should gain 35 to 45 pounds, or about 1 to 1¼ pounds per week. (Figure 7–1 in Chapter 7 shows a pregnancy weight-gain graph for normal-weight women expecting twins.) If underweight prior to pregnancy, a gain of 40 to 50 pounds, or about 1¼ to 1½ pounds a week is advised. Suggested weekly rates of weight gain are adjusted for the shorter pregnancies of women bearing twins. If pregnancy goes beyond thirty-seven weeks, weight gain, rather than a plateau in gain or weight loss, should continue up to delivery.

Vitamin and Mineral Supplements

It is more important that women pregnant with twins eat a good diet and gain weight appropriately than it is to take large amounts of supplements. Only moderate doses of supplemental vitamins and minerals, the same doses as presented in Table 6–1 in Chapter 6, are recommended for women expecting twins. This supplement is recommended for *all* such women. The recommended supplement contains 30 mg of iron for the prevention of iron deficiency anemia. Higher levels of iron or other vitamins and minerals should be taken if a particular need for the nutrients is identified.

For Women Expecting Triplets

There is little information available about special nutritional considerations for women carrying triplets. It is advised, however, that additional weight be gained (about 10 pounds more than that recommended for twins) and that at least one additional serving from each food group be consumed daily.

~ 11 ~

Nutrition After Pregnancy: Infant Feeding

Food is the first enjoyment of life.

—Lin Yutang

Think of this chapter as an owner's manual on infant feeding. (The operational manual on breast-feeding follows in the next chapter.) There is a good deal to be said about infant feeding, but with a new baby in your life or on the way, you probably have too little time to read. Therefore, this chapter focuses on just the facts. It includes a variety of tables for ready reference and highlights information that will help you make the right decisions about nourishing your infant. Answers to questions commonly asked about infant feeding are included at the end of the chapter.

Good Things to Know About Infant Feeding

All newborns, whether breast-fed or bottle-fed, have the same need for nutrients—a need that is greater than it will ever be again. Yet, fulfilling this need requires a very simple diet. Babies thrive on just one food, breast milk or infant formula, for the first four to six months of life. A baby's need for nutrients is a result of his or her rapid growth and development (see Table 11–1).

For the first two months of life, a baby will gain about an ounce a day, or a little less than a pound every two weeks. If growth proceeds on course, a baby's birth weight will triple and her or his length will increase by 50 percent by the end of the first year of

Table 11-1 Growth and Development Characteristics from Birth
Through One Year

Age	Characteristics
First Days of Life	Generally weighs from 7 to 9 pounds, length 19 to 21 inches. Head is relatively large and has soft spot on top. Startles and sneezes easily. Jaw may tremble. May hiccough and spit up.
One Month	Has regained weight lost after birth and more. Lifts head briefly when placed on stomach. Whole body moves when touched or lifted.
Four Months	Weight nearly doubled. Has grown three to four inches. Follows objects with eyes. Reaches toward objects with both hands. Plays with fingers. Puts fingers and objects into mouth. Holds head up steadily, though back needs support. Attempts to roll over. Sleeps six to seven hours at night.
Eight Months	Gains in weight and height are less rapid, appetite has decreased. Rolls over; stands up with help; sits up; hitches self along the floor. Reaches for, grasps, and examines objects with hands, eyes, and mouth. Has one or two teeth. Takes two naps a day. Loses some "baby fat" as activity increases.
Twelve Months	Usually has tripled birth weight and increased length by 50 percent. Grasps and releases objects with fingers. Holds spoon, but uses it poorly.

life. This is an enormous rate of growth. If that pace were to continue, a five-year-old child would weigh about a ton and stand more than 13 feet tall!

How much a baby will want to eat depends on her or his rate of growth. Babies grow in spurts, rather than at a gradual, constant pace. They will be noticeably more hungry right before a growth spurt. One very common pregrowth period occurs for most babies when they are fourteen to twenty-eight days old. So don't be shocked if your baby seems to want to eat all the time during those two weeks.

Because a baby naturally adjusts his or her appetite to the level needed for growth, you should feed your newborn whenever she or he is hungry. Feeding babies "by the clock" may lead to overeating or undereating. Wait until your baby is nine months old or more before you attempt to fit his or her meals into your family's schedule. By nine months, most babies can adjust to eating meals with the rest of the family. They will still need snacks whenever they are hungry, however.

Because babies have a great need for nutrients and small stomachs, they get hungry often. During the first few weeks, your baby will probably want to eat every two or three hours, or eight to twelve times a day. At each feeding, she or he will drink about 2 or 3 ounces of breast milk or formula. By your baby's second month, the interval between his or her demands to be fed may stretch to three or four hours. By nine months, most babies need to eat only five to seven times per day. These and other developmental considerations related to infant feeding are summarized in Table 11–2.

Feedings should be followed by burpings. Babies swallow air along with their breast milk or formula. After a meal, they receive considerable relief and comfort from a few gentle pats on the back.

Recognizing a Hungry Baby

Because babies cry or become fussy for a variety of reasons, recognizing when a baby is hungry can be difficult. Hungry babies, however, feed with enthusiasm. They shut out the rest of the world while they are eating. Hungry babies start feeding with clenched fists, suck eagerly, and forget their discomfort as soon as they start to eat. A baby who really wants something other than food will suck on the bottle or breast halfheartedly and will be easily distracted.

It is also important to recognize when a baby has had enough to eat. Accept the baby's decision that she or he is no longer hungry. Don't coax the baby into eating more or finishing the last ounce of formula or bits of food left on the plate. Healthy babies will eat when they are hungry and stop eating when they are full.

Table 11–2 Developmental Considerations Related to Infant Feeding

Age	Skills
Newborn	"Rooting reflex" present (will find nipple if placed near breast); sucks and swallows liquids; "gag reflex" (will gag if solid foods are placed near back of tongue); eats every two to three hours.
Two months	May begin to sleep longer during the night; fewer night feedings needed.
Three months	Gag reflex relaxes; enzymes needed to digest solid foods mature; kidney and digestive tract matures (baby is getting ready for solid foods).
Four months	Able to swallow nonliquid foods; eats seven to eight times per day; can hold objects between palm and fingers.
Five months	Puts things in mouth with hands; can form a bolus (a ball of food) and move it from the front to the back of the mouth and swallow it.
Six months	Chewing skills begin to develop.
Seven months	Can grasp food with fingers; able to chew and swallow lumpy foods and finger foods; sucks from a cup; can pick up cup but not able to put it down; holds own bottle.
Eight months	Feeds self from bottle (tips it up, if needed).
Nine to twelve months	Chewing and swallowing steadily improve; able to handle spoon, cup better; eats five to seven times a day.

Infant Feeding Recommendations

Recommendations for feeding infants are primarily based on energy and nutrient needs, the developmental readiness of infants for solid foods, and the prevention of food allergies. Infant feeding recommendations also include a large educational component. Many of the lessons infants learn about food and eating make an impression that lasts a lifetime. Later food habits and preferences, appetite, and food intake regulation are each influenced by early learning experiences. Table 11–3 provides a plan for teaching your infant the right lessons about food and eating.

Feeding Infants in the First Six Months of Life

An age-appropriate schedule for the introduction of foods into infants' diets is shown in Table 11–4.

Infants should be breast-fed or given iron fortified infant formula for the first twelve months of life, and semisolid foods should be started between four and six months. Nonallergenic, easy-to-digest foods, such as rice cereal and strained fruits and vegetables should be introduced first. The introduction of foods most likely to cause allergic or other adverse reactions should be delayed until babies are at least six months old. Infants with a family history of food allergies, however, may benefit if these foods are not introduced until after the first year. Cow's milk, soy milk, wheat products, nuts (including peanut butter), eggs, and shellfish most commonly cause allergies. Food intolerance reactions, such as skin rash or diarrhea, may be associated with the early introduction of corn, prune juice, orange juice, chocolate, and strawberries. A variety of other foods may also cause food intolerance reactions.

Do Solid Foods Help the Baby Sleep Longer?

It was once thought that solid foods should be offered to infants within the first month or two of life. Although such young infants are unable to swallow much of the food offered (most of it ends up on their faces and bibs), or to digest completely what they do

Table 11–3 Tips for Teaching Infants the Right Lessons About Food and Eating

---

1. Infants learn to eat a variety of healthy foods by being offered an assortment of wholesome choices. There are NO inborn mechanisms that direct babies to select a nutritious diet.

2. Infants must be allowed to eat when they are hungry and to stop eating when they are full. Infants, not parents, know when they are hungry or have had enough to eat.

3. Food should be offered in a pleasant environment with positive adult attention.

4. Food should not be used as a reward or punishment, or as a pacifier.

5. Infants or children should never be coerced into eating anything.

6. Food preferences change throughout infancy. Because an infant rejects a food one time doesn't mean that she or he will not accept the food if offered later. Giving a food on a number of occasions often improves acceptance of it. Babies still might not like strong-flavored vegetables until they are older, however.

---

swallow, solid foods were thought to fill the baby up and help him or her sleep through the night. Giving solid foods before the age of four months does not accomplish that. Infants who are fed solids early are no more likely to sleep through the night than are those who start to eat solid foods between four and six months of age. The age at which an infant begins to sleep for six or more hours during the night depends on other factors, including the infant's developmental level and how much she or he has slept during the day. Neither the infant nor the parents are likely to get a good night's sleep for at least four months.

Feeding Infants in the Second Six Months of Life

Strained meats (chicken, turkey, beef, and pork) and legumes (cooked dried beans and peas) are good foods to introduce between six and seven months. By the time an infant is seven months old, he or she is ready to chew or to gum and swallow

Table 11–4 Infant Feeding Recommendations

Age	Feeding Recommendations
Birth through four to six months	Breast-feed or give iron-fortified infant formula only. • Continue breast- or formula-feeding through the first year of life • Breast-fed babies with inadequate exposure to sunshine should be given a vitamin D supplement (200 IU per day)
Four to six months	Introduce rice cereal and then strained, plain fruits and vegetables • Use iron-fortified cereal if baby is breast-fed • Start with small portions (1 to 2 teaspoons) and build up to larger portions (2 to 3 tablespoons) for three meals a day by six months
Six to seven months	Add strained, plain meats and/or legumes; and fruit juices • Breast-fed babies and babies given formula not diluted with fluoridated tap water should be given a fluoride supplement (0.25 mg fluoride per day)
Seven to nine months	Use soft foods that provide some texture (for example, mashed, finely chopped, and lumpy foods) Give finger foods (see Table 11–6)
Nine to twelve months	Offer a variety of mashed and cut-up table foods from family meals
One year	Eggs and whole cow's milk can be introduced after the first twelve months; low-fat milk should not be used until the age of two years or more

foods with a bit of texture. Offering textured foods at this time helps the baby learn to chew and swallow and appears to foster the development of speaking skills. Foods offered should be the consistency of thick soup and contain lumpy pieces of soft food. Although you can purchase baby foods of the right consistency, you can also make them at home using a food mill or food processor. Directions for making baby food at home are given in Table 11–5.

Finger foods should also be introduced when the baby is seven months old. Foods offered should be easy to pick up, not require much chewing, and be in small enough pieces so that they can be easily swallowed. A list of good and bad choices for finger foods is given in Table 11–6.

By nine months of age, infants are ready for mashed and finely cut-up foods. Infants graduate to adult-type foods toward the end of the first year of life. Although most foods still need to be mashed or cut up into small pieces, one-year-olds are able to eat the same types of foods as the rest of the family. They can drink from a cup and nearly feed themselves with a spoon. Infants have come a long way in twelve months!

Do Infants Need Vitamin or Mineral Supplements?

Two situations call for the use of supplements during infancy. Breast-fed infants and infants receiving formula from a concentrate not diluted with fluoridated water need fluoride supplements after six months of age. Since breast milk contains a low amount of vitamin D, breast-fed infants not exposed regularly to sunshine should receive 5 μg (200 IU) vitamin D as a daily supplement. Babies who are exposed to sunshine thirty minutes per week while in diapers only, or two hours per week if only the head is exposed, make enough vitamin D in their skin. Care should be taken to ensure the baby isn't overexposed to sunshine. Sunbathing infants in the indirect rays of the sun in the morning and late afternoon is best in the summer months. Periods of direct exposure to sunshine without sunscreen should be brief, ten minutes or less at a time.

Table 11–5 Making Baby Foods at Home

Equipment needed: A blender or baby-food mill and a strainer.
Set-up: Clean all utensils, equipment, and counter surfaces thoroughly.
Wash hands with soap and water.

PREPARATION

Use basic foods that do not contain added sugar, salt, spices, margarine, butter,
or other additives. After the infant is seven months old, make the food a bit
lumpy, but still soft.

FRUITS	Use clean and ripe fruits. Remove all skin, seeds, and cores (or use canned fruits). Puree in blender or food mill thoroughly. (Cook hard fruits like apples first.) Mash if fruit is soft enough.
Examples:	Mashed bananas; applesauce; pureed apricots, pears, and peaches.
VEGETABLES	Clean thoroughly. Remove stems and any tough skin or seeds. Boil or steam until soft. Puree and serve lukewarm.
Examples:	Pureed green beans, peas, squash, carrots, and potatoes.
MEATS	Cook the meat thoroughly. Trim off fat, skin, and gristle. Blend or grind meat with enough water to make a puree (generally ½ cup water to 1 cup cooked meat).
Examples:	Pork, chicken, fish, beef, lamb, turkey.
JUICES	Use frozen or bottled apple, cranberry, and grape juice. Reconstitute frozen juices according to directions on the container. Strain juice if needed. Avoid "fruit drinks."

STORAGE

Freeze extra servings in a tightly covered ice-cube tray or other airtight
container, or store tightly covered in refrigerator for no more than three days.
Do not thaw and refreeze.

Discard any leftovers in the baby's dish. When the spoon used to feed the
child contacts the food, bacteria is introduced that may cause the food to
spoil while stored.

Table 11–6 Good and Bad Choices for Finger Foods

Good Choices	Bad Choices
cracker pieces	raisins
melba toast (zwieback)	seeds
soft fruit pieces	hard candy
Cheerios	hot dog or sausage pieces
soft pieces of vegetables	popcorn, granola
soft macaroni pieces	grapes, blueberries
small pieces of soft cheese	nuts, peanut butter
	raw vegetables
	corn
	chips

Questions About Infant Feeding

Q. *What's the best infant formula to give my baby?*

A. Commercially available cow's milk–based formulas are recommended and all brands are similar in composition. In fact, there are standards for formula composition to which all manufacturers must adhere. Consequently, any formula will provide complete nutrition for your baby. It is best to use an iron-fortified formula. Babies need the extra iron to build up their iron stores.

Q. *Is bottle feeding as good as breast-feeding?*

A. Breast-feeding is the number one choice for infant feeding. It is not, however, best for women who do not want to breast-feed. Infant formulas are an appropriate alternative to breast-feeding for women who would feel forced into breast-feeding or for other reasons would not be able to breast-feed successfully. Although there are benefits to breast milk, the benefits don't apply if the mother is not a willing participant and breast-feeding is continued even though it is not going well.

Q. *Should I heat up the milk before I give it to my baby?*

A. Most babies don't have a temperature preference. You may want to take the chill off a cold bottle of formula by running warm water over it. It is better to give the baby milk that is cool rather than too warm. Heating milk in the microwave can make it too hot, and is not recommended.

Q. *Is it okay to put the baby to bed with a bottle at night?*

A. The fluid that drips into the baby's mouth after she or he falls asleep promotes tooth decay and ear infections. Therefore, a baby should not be put to bed with a bottle.

Q. *Is it okay to encourage my baby to drink the last few ounces of milk in the bottle?*

A. No. You should quit feeding the baby when she or he has lost interest in eating.

Q. *Does my baby need vitamin supplements?*

A. Healthy infants born at term do not need multivitamin supplements.

Q. *Is it okay to mix rice cereal with formula in the bottle?*

A. The practice is not recommended. Eating from a spoon helps develop infant feeding skills.

Q. *When can I use cow's milk instead of formula?*

A. After the first year. Introduction of cow's milk too soon can lead to blood loss from the baby's gastrointestinal tract.

Q. *What foods are most likely to cause allergies in infants?*

A. Many types of foods can cause adverse reactions in infants. The most common allergy-causing foods are cow's milk, soy milk, wheat products, nuts (including peanut butter), eggs, and seafood.

Q. *Do I have to sterilize the bottles and nipples?*

A. No, just make sure they are cleaned thoroughly with soap and water and rinsed well.

Q. *How do I know if the baby is getting enough formula?*

A. During the first month, most babies drink about 3 ounces of formula at each feeding, or 20 to 24 ounces in a twenty-four-hour period. In the second month, usual intake is 26 to 28 ounces, and in the third month, 28 to 36 ounces. The baby's weight gain is also a good indicator of the adequacy of food intake.

Q. *Why aren't baby foods introduced until four to six months?*

A. The introduction of semisolid foods at four to six months is recommended because infants are not developmentally ready to swallow foods, and their digestive systems are too immature to process them before that time. Introducing solids early also promotes the development of food allergies.

Q. *Is goat's milk better for the baby than cow's milk?*

A. Goat's milk is not better than cow's milk, but neither one is recommended until after age one. Both have levels of protein and minerals that are too high for humans during the first year of life.

Q. *I've heard babies shouldn't be given honey. Is that true?*

A. Babies should not be given unpasteurized honey because it may cause botulism in infants. Pasteurized honey is safe, but babies don't need sweets anyway.

Q. *Should I cut back on the amount of food I give my baby if he is getting too fat?*

A. No. Babies are normally fat. They should be allowed to decide when they are hungry and when they've had enough to eat. Babies begin to thin down after they start to crawl and become more physically active.

⌒ 12 ⌒

Nutrition After Pregnancy: Breast-feeding

Nourish the mother to nourish the baby.

N ext to every well-nourished, breast-fed baby is a well-nourished mother. She is ideally suited for making the perfect food for her infant. Breast milk provides infants with optimal nutrition and much more. It gives infants regular, oral vaccinations against common diseases of childhood including ear infections, diarrhea, and respiratory infections. It is easier for babies to digest than formulas. Breast-fed babies are less likely to experience food allergies, diabetes, and certain types of cancer during childhood. Breast milk is the best source of nutrition for most preterm babies. Since the taste of breast milk varies with the mother's diet, breast-fed babies experience a wider variety of tastes than do formula-fed infants. In addition, the unique assortment of fatty acids in breast milk enhances brain development and intelligence. If breast milk were manufactured by a pharmaceutical company, it would be considered a miracle drug. Breast milk is a gift brought to us by Mother Nature that everyone can afford.

Breast-feeding benefits women as well as infants. When infants breast-feed, the hormone oxytocin is released and stimulates the contraction of uterine muscles. The contraction of the uterus helps stop bleeding caused by the detachment of the placenta from the wall of the uterus. (This effect of breast-feeding can be quite noticeable. During the first few days after delivery, women can often feel the uterus contract while breast-feeding.) Women who breast-feed lose an average of 4 to 5 pounds more within the first year after delivery than women who do not breast-feed. Breast-feeding appears to reduce the risk of developing breast and ovarian cancer later in life. The longer women breast-feed or the more infants that are breast-fed, the less likely women are to develop these disorders. An additional and important advantage of breast-feeding is that it is an enjoyable experience. Breast-feeding can be a great source of satisfaction and pleasure.

The benefits of breast-feeding for both mother and baby make it the clear choice for infant feeding. Yet, due to the demands of work shortly after delivery, a disinterest in breast-feeding, or health problems, breast-feeding may not be best for all women and infants. Women who feel that they have been coerced into breast-feeding and will never feel comfortable with it probably should not breast-feed. It may be difficult to do successfully if your heart is not in it.

If you are uncertain whether you should breast- or formula-feed, knowing more about how breast-feeding works may help you make the decision. You can also consider the following fifteen other reasons for breast-feeding:

1. Milk container is easy to clean.
2. Breast milk is a renewable resource.
3. There's no packaging to discard.
4. Breast milk comes in an attractive container.
5. The temperature of breast milk is always perfect right out of the container.
6. Breast milk tastes real good.
7. There are no leftovers.
8. You don't have to go to the kitchen in the middle of the night to get it ready.
9. It takes just seconds to get a meal ready.
10. There's no bottle to repeatedly pick up off the floor.
11. The price is right.
12. The meal comes in a perfect serving size.
13. Meals and snacks are easy to bring along on a trip or outing.
14. Feeding units come in an assortment of decorative colors and sizes.
15. One food makes a complete meal.

If you have decided to breast-feed, this chapter will give you information that can be used to help the experience go smoothly. It covers facts about how breast-feeding works and how you know when it's going well, and dietary recommendations for breast-feeding women. Questions commonly asked about breast-feeding are answered at the end of the chapter.

How Breast-feeding Works

A woman's body begins to prepare for breast-feeding during pregnancy. It does so by depositing fat in breast tissue and by expanding the network of blood vessels that infiltrate the cells of the breast. Ducts that channel milk from the milk-producing cells forward to the nipple also mature.

Hormonal changes that occur at delivery signal milk production to begin. Since delivery rather than length of pregnancy initiates milk production, breast milk is available for infants born prematurely.

Milk produced by women during the first few days after delivery is different from the milk produced later. The early milk is called *colostrum* and contains a higher level of antibodies, protein, and minerals than does "mature" milk, or the milk produced when the baby is about three or four days old. Colostrum is a concentrated source of preventive medicine. It provides infants with a boost of infection-fighting antibodies for their entrance from a germ-free environment into one that is germ filled. Colostrum is thicker than mature milk, and has a yellowish color.

Mature milk comes in two types: *foremilk* and *hindmilk*. Foremilk represents about a third of the available milk supply, while hindmilk makes up the rest. Present in the ducts that lead from the milk-producing cells to the nipple, foremilk is readily available to the infant. It contains less fat and protein, and therefore, fewer calories than hindmilk.

Hindmilk is stored in the milk producing cells of the breast. Unlike foremilk, hindmilk is not automatically available to the infant. It is released by oxytocin, the same hormone that signals the uterus to contract during the first few days after delivery. Oxytocin causes the milk-producing cells to contract and thereby release the hindmilk. This process is commonly referred to as the *letdown reflex*. The milk-releasing effect of oxytocin is so powerful that milk is actually ejected from the breast. If the hindmilk is not released, the infant will not get enough milk, will be hungry most of the time, and may grow and develop poorly. A number of conditions can interfere with the release of oxytocin and, therefore, the release of hindmilk during breast-feeding. The failure of the letdown reflex is a major cause of breast-feeding failure.

Factors Affecting the Letdown Reflex

The letdown reflex can be initiated by either physical or psychological factors. It is commonly started by the physical sensation of the infant sucking at the nipple but can also occur when a mother hears an infant cry or even when the thought "it's time for a feeding" enters her mind. The physical or psychological stimulus signals a part of the brain to release oxytocin into the bloodstream. When it reaches its target, the milk-producing cells contract and eject their content of milk.

Certain forms of physical and psychological stimuli can prevent the letdown reflex. Stress, pain, anxiety, and other distractions can block the release of oxytocin. If a woman is in pain or if she is pressed for time, for example, the letdown reflex may not occur. When this happens often enough, women may think they don't have enough milk and may decide to switch to formula feeding. In these cases, a lack of milk isn't the problem; the failure to experience the letdown reflex is. Breast-feeding in comfortable and relaxed surroundings, and the uninhibited enjoyment of breast-feeding, help foster the letdown reflex.

Breast Milk Production

While an infant is consuming one meal, she or he is ordering the next. The pressure produced inside the breast by the infant's sucking and the emptying of the breast during a feeding cause the hormone prolactin to be released from special cells in the brain. Prolactin stimulates the production of milk. The breasts will produce as much milk as the infant consumes. It generally takes about two hours for the milk-producing cells to make enough milk for the infant's next feeding. An important exception to the two-hour refill time, however, occurs when an infant is about to enter a growth spurt and eats more to prepare for it.

Infants, like children and adolescents, grow in spurts and not at a constant rate. In preparation for a growth spurt, hunger increases and the intake of breast milk may double. The first noticeable growth spurt generally occurs between fourteen and twenty-eight days of age. The increase in breast milk intake associated with a pending growth spurt lengthens the time it takes to produce a refill in milk supply. Instead of two hours, it may take twenty-four hours for breast milk production to catch up with demand. This means that for about a day, infants will want to feed often and will not have their hunger completely satisfied. Although women may spend much of their day breast-feeding an infant who is entering a growth spurt, as long as the infant is allowed to breast-feed as often as desired, production will catch up with the baby's need for milk. Adding formula to the baby's diet will decrease production because the baby will consume less breast milk.

Ensuring That the Baby Is Getting Enough Breast Milk

Unlike bottle feeding, there is no way for a breast-feeding woman to know how much food the baby has consumed. Breast-feeding women must make assumptions about whether a baby is getting enough to eat by signals the infant sends out. Babies who regain their birth weight by two weeks, suck vigorously, are hungry no more often than every two to four hours, and who are gaining weight at an appropriate rate are most likely getting enough breast milk. Unfortunately, when babies don't get enough milk over the course of days or weeks, they may not send out signals that indicate that this is happening. Young infants who fail to consume sufficient milk may become quiet, sullen, and sleep a lot. When offered the breast, they may suck weakly and not appear to be hungry. The lack of food has zapped their energy, and since they may not complain, it is hard to know there is anything wrong.

If you are concerned your baby isn't getting enough breast milk, check out the following:

- Is the baby's rate of weight gain okay? (You may have to check with your health care provider to find out. Few women have an infant scale at home.)
- Are there fewer than six to eight wet diapers a day? Does the baby have fewer than three to five bowel movements daily? There should be at least this many.
- Is the inside of the baby's mouth dry? It should be moist.
- Can you hear the baby swallow milk while feeding? Swallowing noises should be audible.
- Is the baby's suck weak? It should be strong, especially at the beginning of the feeding.
- Is the duration of feeding short, or less than a few minutes? Babies usually consume 70 percent of the total milk within five minutes of beginning breast-feeding, and 90 percent by ten minutes.
- Is the frequency of feeding less than eight times a day? Babies are generally hungry eight to twelve times per day in the early months of life.
- Are you experiencing the letdown reflex? Many women can feel the letdown reflex as a prickly sensation in the nipples within the first minute of breast-feeding. You know you have experienced the letdown reflex if milk spurts, rather than drips, from your breast when the baby is removed a minute or so after breast-feeding has begun.

Not all babies displaying one or more of these signs will be consuming too little breast milk. They are warning signs, however, and should be brought to the attention of your health care provider without delay.

Can Breast-fed Babies Be Overfed?

Breast-fed babies, like formula-fed babies, can be overfed. Overfeeding usually results from nursing the baby for the wrong reason. Babies often receive comfort from sucking on a breast when they are tired, anxious, frustrated, or simply feeling the need to suck. Try a pacifier, some cuddling, a change of diapers, or a burping before you offer your breast to a baby who you suspect is not hungry.

How Long Should Breast-feeding Continue?

No one knows what the best length of breast-feeding is in terms of infant health. It has been observed over time, however, that women in most cultures generally breast-feed for six months to two years. Milk-producing animals, such as dogs, cats, mice, and rats, tend to breast-feed for about the same length of time as pregnancy. Rats, for example, take about twenty-one days to produce the litter and breast-feed their young for approximately the first twenty-one days after birth. Whether nine months is the best length of time for breast-feeding humans is debatable. However, it appears that breast-feeding for six months to a year may represent an appropriate range. It is recommended that infants be exclusively breast-fed for the first four to six months of life. Any duration of breast-feeding is better than none, however.

Weaning Babies Off Breast Milk

Breast milk production will continue as long as an infant feeds at the breast. Milk production decreases when other foods are given, when the intervals between feedings lengthen, and when the breasts aren't completely emptied after feedings. It ceases altogether when the infant stops breast-feeding.

Breast-feeding Dilemmas

Ninety-nine percent of women who want to breast-feed are physically able to do so. The psychological disposition of the mother, and a supportive environment, are the key factors involved in successful breast-feeding. Breast-feeding requires time, patience, understanding, and a sense of humor. It is a learning process for both mother and baby.

The greatest period of adjustment to breast-feeding generally occurs during the first seven to ten days after delivery. It is not uncommon for problems with breast-feeding to arise during this time, but with appropriate guidance and support, difficulties can usually be quickly resolved. The best way to handle problems with breast-feeding is by obtaining professional guidance and support from a knowledgeable individual. Some problems can be resolved by a phone call to your health care provider, while others are best mended by a lactation consultant. Several resources for breast-feeding guidance and support are listed at the end of this chapter. Do not hesitate to take advantage of the knowledge and skills of people who know how to fix breast-feeding difficulties.

Dietary Recommendations for Breast-feeding Women

An adequate and balanced diet is needed by breast-feeding women for their own health and stamina, to replenish nutrient stores called upon during pregnancy, and to produce an ample supply of breast milk. For breast-feeding, you "nourish the baby by nourishing the mother."

Calorie and Nutrient Needs

A woman's need for calories during breast-feeding is around 25 percent higher than it is for nonpregnant women. Since energy supplied from fat stores contribute to meeting this need, not all the extra energy has to come from the diet. In general, a diet that provides about 500 calories more per day than before pregnancy meets a woman's energy needs for breast milk production. It also allows for loss in body weight of approximately one-half pound per week.

The Recommended Dietary Allowances (RDAs) for breast-feeding women are between 25 and 67 percent higher than normal. (Table 12–1 lists the RDAs for breast-feeding.)

As is the case for pregnancy, proportionately higher amounts of nutrients and calories are required for breast-feeding, and that adds up to the need for a nutrient-dense diet. The extra water that is needed for breast-feeding is generally obtained without any special effort. Women simply need to drink enough fluids to satisfy thirst.

Effects of Maternal Diet on Breast Milk Composition

Milk-producing cells in the breast are supplied with the raw materials they need to manufacture milk from the mother's blood. For most substances, what ends up in the mother's blood reflects what she consumed. Consequently, the composition of breast milk varies somewhat depending on the mother's diet. For other substances, the amount that enters breast milk is regulated within the milk-producing cells and the levels remain fairly constant regardless of maternal diet.

Table 12–1 Recommended Dietary Allowances (RDAs) for Breast-feeding

Nutrient	RDA
Protein	65 g
Vitamin A	1,300 RE (6,500 IU)
Vitamin D	10 µg (400 IU)
Vitamin E	12 mg (36 IU)
Vitamin K	95 µg
Vitamin C	70 mg
Thiamin	1.6 mg
Riboflavin	1.8 mg
Niacin	20 mg NE
Vitamin B$_6$	2.1 mg
Folate	280 µg
Vitamin B$_{12}$	2.6 µg
Calcium	1,200 mg
Phosphorus	1,200 mg
Magnesium	355 mg
Iron	15 mg
Zinc	19 mg
Iodine	200 µg
Selenium	75 µg

Source: National Academy of Sciences, 1989.

Milk-producing cells enforce quality control processes that regulate the amount of carbohydrate, protein, fat, and many minerals in breast milk. They also regulate the amount of milk produced when maternal caloric intake is too low. Rather than dilute the energy content of milk in response to a low-calorie diet, the volume of milk decreases.

The vitamin and mineral content of breast milk can be affected by maternal diet. The amount of thiamin, vitamin C, and vitamin B_{12} in breast milk, for example, varies based on the types of foods and supplements that the mother ingests. Thiamin deficiency (beriberi), iodine deficiency, cretinism, vitamin D deficiency (rickets), and vitamin B_{12} deficiency (pernicious anemia) have been diagnosed in infants breast-fed by mothers lacking sufficient nutrient levels.

A Good Diet for Breast-feeding

The energy and nutrients needed to sustain the health of women who breast-feed and for the production of the perfect food for infants can be obtained by consuming the variety of foods recommended in Table 12–2.

If you are not sure whether your diet contains the appropriate assortment of foods, evaluate it as you did in Chapter 5. A form for recording your usual diet is given in Table 12–3.

You may need to consume the lower number of servings recommended for some of the food groups if weight loss is desired, or more servings if weight is being lost too quickly.

Weight Loss During Breast-feeding

Weight loss that exceeds 1½ pounds per week, even in women with a good supply of fat stores, can reduce the amount of breast milk produced. Consequently, weight loss should be limited to about 2 pounds per month after the first month postpartum if women are near normal weight and 4 pounds per month if they are overweight. Liquid diets or diet pills are not recommended for breast-feeding women.

Table 12–2 Evaluating Your Diet for Breast-feeding

Food Guide Pyramid group	Standard serving sizes	Recommended servings per day	Number of servings I had	Difference in servings
1. Bread, cereal, rice, and pasta	bread, 1 slice cereal, 1 cup hot cereal, ½ cup bagel, ½ rice or pasta, ½ cup tortilla, 1	6–11		
2. Vegetables	raw or cooked, ½ cup leafy, 1 cup juice, ¾ cup	3–5		
3. Fruits	fresh, 1 piece canned, ½ cup juice, ¾ cup	2–4		
4. Milk, yogurt, and cheese	milk, 1 cup soy milk, 1 cup yogurt, 1 cup cottage cheese, ½ cup cheese, 1½ ounces	4		
5. Meat, poultry, fish, dry beans, eggs, and nuts	meat, 3 ounces dried beans, ½ cup tofu, ½ cup eggs, 2 peanut butter, 4 tablespoons	3		
6. Fats, oils, and sweets	fats and oils, 2 teaspoons sweets, 1 ounce	limited		

Table 12–3 Usual Diet Recording Form

| Time of Day | DAY 1 | | | DAY 2 | |
	What I Ate and Drank	Amount		What I Ate and Drank	Amount
Example:					
Noon	Chef's salad:			Vegetarian lasagna:	
	Romaine	2 cups		pasta	1 cup
	turkey	1 ounce		tomato sauce	½ cup
	ham	1 ounce		zucchini	¼ cup
	cheese	1 ounce		cheese	1 ounce
	iced tea	1½ cups		milk	1 cup
Morning					
Midmorning					
Noon					
Afternoon					
Evening					
Late evening					

Maternal Diet and Infant Colic

The various causes of colic aren't known with certainty and that makes it a difficult problem to treat. However, certain foods in a woman's diet appear to be one of the causes of colic symptoms. Cow's milk, chocolate, onions, brussels sprouts, broccoli, cabbage, and cauliflower in the mother's diet have been related to the development of colic symptoms in infants.

Is Alcohol Okay?

Alcohol in a woman's diet appears in breast milk. Oddly enough, beer or wine is sometimes recommended to women to "help them relax" before breast-feeding. Although one or two alcohol-containing beverages per day appear to pose no harm to the breast-fed infant, heavy drinking during breast-feeding can expose infants to levels of alcohol that may harm their development. The development of the brains and nervous systems of infants born to chronic, heavy drinkers appears to be retarded.

Environmental Contaminants in Breast Milk

Environmental contaminants such as organochlorinated pesticide residues, polychlorinated biphenyls (PCBs), and mercury are transferred into breast milk. Many environmental contaminants are fat soluble and if consumed will be stored in a woman's fat tissue. When her fat stores are broken down for use in breast milk, the contaminants stored in fat enter the milk. The ingestion of fish from the contaminated waters of Lake Ontario and Lake Michigan have been related to abnormally high levels of PCBs in breast milk. Other, localized outbreaks of contamination of breast milk have been reported. Clearly, women should not eat fish from contaminated waterways. Many lakes and rivers have signs posted that indicate the water is contaminated and that fish from that water should not be consumed. Your local health department can advise you on sources of contaminated water in your area. However, most often a woman's exposure to toxic substances from the environment is low enough as not to harm the baby. The benefits of breast-feeding far outweigh risks associated with environmental toxin exposure for the vast majority of breast-fed infants.

Are Vitamin and Mineral Supplements Needed?

Vitamin and mineral supplements are not needed by healthy women who consume an adequate diet while breast-feeding. Vegans and women who do not consume a source of vitamin D or have little direct exposure to sunshine should take a vitamin D supplement of 10 μg (400 IU) per day. Women with low intakes of vitamin D should also take care to eat enough calcium-rich foods. Vegans should also be sure they are getting enough vitamin B_{12}.

Breast-fed babies may need a 5 μg (200 IU) vitamin D supplement daily if they receive little exposure to sunlight (less than thirty minutes per week with just diapers on or two hours per week if only the head is exposed). Infants should be prescribed a 0.25 mg fluoride supplement after six months of age.

Questions About Breast-feeding

If your questions about breast-feeding haven't been answered so far in this chapter, read on. You may find the answers you are looking for in this section.

Q. Should I supplement with formula if I'm concerned that my baby isn't getting enough breast milk?

A. It's not a good idea to give a breast-fed baby formula, especially during the first few weeks. Use of formula leads to decreased production of breast milk and a dependence on formula. Allowing the baby to breast-feed on demand (which will be eight to twelve times per day in the first few months) results in a production of breast milk that matches the amount the baby needs. If your baby doesn't eat often enough, try waking him or her up and feeding every few hours. If you are concerned your baby is not getting enough breast milk, and one or more of the conditions previously listed in the section, "Ensuring That the Baby Is Getting Enough Breast Milk" is present, seek the advice of your health care provider or a lactation consultant without delay.

Q. *Some days my baby seems particularly hungry and wants to eat all the time. Does this mean I'm not making enough milk?*

A. Your baby is probably preparing for a growth spurt. Your milk supply will catch up with the baby's need for milk within twenty-four hours. Keep feeding frequently to help build up your milk supply.

Babies also have a need to suck aside from their need for food. If the baby wants to be at the breast to be soothed by sucking, a pacifier may do. If a baby is hungry, he or she won't be soothed by a pacifier for long.

Q. *My baby developed jaundice shortly after birth. Should I stop breast-feeding until it goes away?*

A. In an otherwise healthy newborn, it is best to increase the frequency of breast-feeding rather than to stop it. Increasing the frequency of breast-feeding helps cure the jaundice.

Q. *I've developed a breast infection (mastitis). Should I continue to breast-feed?*

A. Yes, if the infection is mild. Antibiotics used to treat mastitis are generally safe for the baby and draining the affected breasts of milk will relieve pressure in the breast. Breast milk is still sterile—it is not affected or contaminated by the infection.

Q. *Are there foods I should avoid in my diet because they may give my baby colic?*

A. Colic, or repeated bouts of crying with gas, cramps, and irritability, can be due to a number of causes, including components of the breast-feeding mother's diet. Eliminating the intake of cow's milk, yogurt, cheese, chocolate, onions, and cruciferous vegetables (broccoli, brusselss sprouts, onions, garlic, cauliflower) may relieve the symptoms of colic in some babies. Babies usually outgrow colic by about four months of age.

Q. *Can I remain a vegetarian and breast-feed?*

A. Yes. Make sure you're getting enough calcium, vitamin D, and vitamin B_{12} from your diet or supplements.

Q. *Does what I eat affect the quality of my breast milk?*

A. Yes, in several ways. A healthy diet is the best ingredient for the manufacture of breast milk. Diets that are inadequate in calories may lead to a reduced production of breast milk, and those deficient in vitamins can cause reduced breast milk content of vitamins. The best way to nourish a breast-fed baby is to nourish the mother.

Q. *What is the best way to store breast milk?*

A. Breast milk expressed into a sanitary container can be safely stored in the refrigerator for several days or in the freezer for several months.

Q. *How many extra calories do I need for breast-feeding?*

A. About 500 extra calories, or the amount that doesn't lead to excessively high rates of weight loss or to unneeded weight gain.

Q. *How long should I breast-feed?*

A. Breast-feeding is recommended for the first year of life, but many women happily continue breast-feeding beyond a year. Any duration of breast-feeding is better than none.

Q. *Will I lose weight faster if I breast-feed?*

A. Most women who breast-feed lose 4 to 5 pounds more in the first year after delivery than women who do not breast-feed. Weight-loss results are inconsistent, however, and some women who breast-feed gain weight postpartum. Whether you lose or gain weight depends on energy balance, or if you are expending more calories through breast-feeding and physical activity than you are taking in through food.

Q. *Why is breast-feeding better than formula feeding?*

A. Breast-feeding is better for the baby because of the disease resistance, bone-building, and superior central nervous system development that occurs in babies given breast milk. The composition of breast milk is different and superior to that of infant formulas. With that said, however, breast-feeding is not best for every woman or baby. If breast-feeding is not desired or does not work out for some reason, infant formulas are appropriate.

Q. *Are there any benefits of breast-feeding for the mother?*
A. Yes, there are. Breast-feeding after delivery helps stop uterine bleeding by contracting the uterus. Breast-feeding exclusively helps with child spacing and weight loss. It reduces the risk that women will later develop breast or ovarian cancer.

Q. *Will it harm my baby if I breast-feed while pregnant?*
A. There are no studies that indicate that breast-feeding during pregnancy is harmful.

Q. *Are there any foods I should eat or avoid while breast-feeding?*
A. There are no special foods you should eat. Limiting alcohol intake to one or two drinks per day (if any) and coffee intake to three or four cups a day is recommended. If your baby develops colic, you may want to take cow's milk, chocolate, onions, broccoli, brusselss sprouts, cauliflower, and cabbage out of your diet to see if the colic improves. A variety of other foods from tomatoes to peanut butter may cause skin rashes or other symptoms in your baby. Don't eat the suspected foods.

Babies are much less likely to develop colic after four months of age. At that time, you can reintroduce any foods you may be avoiding because of colic or the threat of it.

Q. *My breasts are small. Can I still make enough milk?*
A. Yes. Milk production doesn't depend on breast size. Women with breasts of all sizes have the parts they need to provide sufficient milk for the baby.

Q. *Should I "force fluids" during breast-feeding?*
A. Breast-feeding women are advised to drink to satisfy their thirst. Drinking a lot of fluids won't increase breast milk volume.

Q. *Should I breast-feed if I want to lose weight quickly after delivery?*
A. If you lose weight too quickly after delivery, you may not be able

to breast-feed. Rapid weight loss during breast-feeding decreases milk volume. If you plan to go on a very low-calorie diet after pregnancy, be prepared to supplement breast milk with infant formula.

Q. *Should I make sure I eat enough protein for breast-feeding?*

A. The RDA for protein for breast-feeding women is 65 grams per day. You can get that much easily by following the diet recommended for breast-feeding (see Table 12–3 in this chapter). Consuming three glasses of milk and two 3-ounce servings of meat per day by themselves provide about 65 grams of protein. Most women consume ample amounts of protein from their normal diets while breast-feeding.

Q. *Is caffeine safe for my baby?*

A. Caffeine does enter breast milk from the mother's diet. Several cups of coffee a day, however, does not appear to be harmful to the baby.

———————

This discussion of breast-feeding brings this book to an end. The advantages of good nutrition do not end with this page, however. Keep up your interest in nutrition!

⌐ Appendix A ⌐

Recipes for Good Eating

What sort of recipes do you keep on file or tucked inside your favorite cookbook? Are they delicious as well as nutritious? If you have an insufficient assortment of such recipes, try these out. They have been designed and tested by the dietitians at Nutrition Plus, Inc., of Minneapolis, Minnesota. Both menus with recipes and single recipes for every course and social occasion are included. Full disclosure about their nutrient contributions is also provided. Your enjoyment of the products of these recipes and your labor will not have to be lessened by a feeling of guilt about what is in them!

Enjoy.

Dinner Menus

COUNTRY BEEF RAGOUT DINNER

Menu	*Suggested Serving Sizes*
Country Beef Ragout*	⅛ of recipe
Cooked egg noodles	1 cup
Tossed salad	1 cup
Low-cal dressing	1 tablespoon
Dinner roll	1
Margarine	1 teaspoon
Skim milk	1 cup
Frozen yogurt	½ cup

* Recipe provided

COUNTRY BEEF RAGOUT (Serves 8)

2 pounds beef stew meat, cut into 1½-inch cubes
3 large onions, each cut into 8 pieces
4 large garlic cloves, crushed
5 tomatoes, quartered
5 tablespoons chopped parsley, divided
1 teaspoon dried thyme leaves
¼ teaspoon pepper
1 cup red Burgundy wine
1 cup water
8 ounces fresh mushrooms, quartered
Wide, flat noodles, cooked

Directions

1. trim excess fat from stew meat. Spray Dutch oven with vegetable spray; add beef cubes and brown over high heat.
2. Add onions and brown lightly; add garlic.

3. Stir in tomatoes, 3 tablespoons parsley, thyme, pepper, red wine and water; bring to a boil.
4. Reduce heat; cover and simmer for 1 hour.
5. Add mushrooms; cover and simmer 60 to 90 minutes, until beef is tender.
6. If desired, simmer uncovered last 10 minutes to reduce liquid.
7. Stir in remaining parsley. Serve ragout over hot cooked noodles.

Composition of Recipe

Serving size: ⅙ of recipe

Calories	307	Zinc (mg)	5.7
Protein (g)	29	Iron (mg)	4.7
Total Fat (g)	14	Vitamin A (IU)	920
Carbohydrate (g)	12	Thiamin (mg)	0.2
Cholesterol (mg)	64	Riboflavin (mg)	0.4
Fiber (g)	2	Niacin (mg)	7.1
Calcium (mg)	46	Vitamin B_6 (mg)	0.5
Magnesium (mg)	53	Folacin (free) (µg)	32
Sodium (mg)	79	Vitamin B_{12} (µg)	2.3
Potassium (mg)	729	Vitamin C (mg)	29

BAKED FISH DINNER

Menu	*Suggested Serving Sizes*
Baked Ocean Perch*	¼ of recipe
Asparagus	4 stalks
Margarine	½ teaspoon
Vinaigrette coleslaw	½ cup
Rye bread	1 slice
Margarine	½ teaspoon
Skim milk	1 cup
Lemon pudding	½ cup

*Recipe provided

Baked Ocean Perch (Serves 4)

1 fresh lemon, thinly sliced
1 medium onion, thinly sliced
¼ teaspoon salt
1 pound ocean perch fillets
1 cup plain low-fat yogurt
1 teaspoon mustard
1 teaspoon paprika

Directions

1. Arrange lemon and onion slices in a lightly greased baking dish.
2. Top with fish fillets and season lightly with salt; cover dish with foil.
3. Bake at 400 degrees for 20 to 25 minutes. Remove foil; turn oven temperature to broil.
4. In a small bowl, blend yogurt, mustard, and paprika; spread over fish.
5. Broil 3 inches from heat for about 5 minutes or until browned.

Composition of Recipe

Serving size: ¼ of recipe

Calories	321	Zinc (mg)	1.8
Protein (g)	26	Iron (mg)	2
Total Fat (g)	17	Vitamin A (IU)	368
Carbohydrate (g)	15	Thiamin (mg)	0.1
Cholesterol (mg)	69	Riboflavin (mg)	0.3
Fiber (g)	0.4	Niacin (mg)	2.3
Calcium (mg)	155	Vitamin B_6 (mg)	0.3
Magnesium (mg)	44	Folacin (free) (µg)	15
Sodium (mg)	375	Vitamin B_{12} (µg)	1.5
Potassium (mg)	529	Vitamin C (mg)	4

CHICKEN CACCIATORE DINNER

Menu	Suggested Serving Sizes
Chicken Cacciatore*	⅙ of recipe
Hot cooked spaghetti	1 cup
Italian Bread	2 pieces
Margarine	1 teaspoon
Skim milk	1 cup
Fruit cocktail	½ cup

*Recipe provided

CHICKEN CACCIATORE (Serves 6)

1½ chickens
2 tablespoons vegetable oil
½ cup flour
2 cups thinly sliced onion rings (2 large)
½ cup chopped green pepper
2 cloves garlic, crushed
4 tomatoes, quartered
1 can (8 ounce) tomato juice
4 ounces fresh mushrooms, sliced
¼ teaspoon salt
½ teaspoon oregano

Directions

1. Wash chicken, pat dry; remove skin and coat chicken with flour.
2. In a Dutch oven or large saucepan, heat oil.
3. Brown chicken in oil; cook over medium heat for 15 to 20 minutes.
4. Remove chicken from saucepan; set aside.
5. Add onion, green pepper, and garlic to saucepan; cook until tender.
6. Add remaining ingredients to saucepan; return chicken to pan.
7. Cover tightly and simmer for 30 to 40 minutes.

Composition of Recipe

Serving size: ⅙ of recipe

Calories	308	Zinc (mg)	2.5
Protein (g)	31	Iron (mg)	2.9
Total Fat (g)	12	Vitamin A (IU)	1360
Carbohydrate (g)	21	Thiamin (mg)	0.2
Cholesterol (mg)	81	Riboflavin (mg)	0.4
Fiber (g)	2.8	Niacin (mg)	11
Calcium (mg)	51	Vitamin B_6 (mg)	0.7
Magnesium (mg)	57	Folacin (free) (µg)	39
Sodium (mg)	377	Vitamin B_{12} (µg)	0.3
Potassium (mg)	762	Vitamin C (mg)	49

TACO SALAD SUPPER

Menu	*Suggested Serving Sizes*
Taco Salad*	⅙ of recipe
Skim milk	1 cup
Sherbet	1 cup

*Recipe provided

TACO SALAD (Serves 6)

1 pound lean ground beef
½ clove garlic, crushed
1 can (4 ounces) mild green chiles, chopped
1 can (16 ounces) tomatoes, undrained
¼ teaspoon salt
⅛ teaspoon pepper
1 head iceberg lettuce, torn into bite-size pieces
⅔ cup grated Cheddar cheese (3 ounces)
3 ounces tortilla chips, crushed
½ cup green onions, chopped
1 tomato, sliced

Directions

1. Sauté beef and garlic until beef is browned. Drain.
2. Add green chiles, canned tomatoes, salt, and pepper, and mix well. Cook uncovered over low heat for 30 minutes.
3. Just before serving, arrange lettuce, cheese, chips, and green onion in a salad bowl. Add meat mixture and toss lightly. Garnish with sliced tomato and serve immediately.

This is also a good main course luncheon salad.

Composition of Recipe

Serving size: ⅙ of recipe

Calories	292	Zinc (mg)	4.6
Protein (g)	23	Iron (mg)	3.5
Total Fat (g)	15	Vitamin A (IU)	1560
Carbohydrate (g)	17	Thiamin (mg)	0.2
Cholesterol (mg)	49	Riboflavin (mg)	0.3
Fiber (g)	2.7	Niacin (mg)	4.6
Calcium (mg)	287	Vitamin B_6 (mg)	0.5
Magnesium (mg)	53	Folacin (free) (µg)	38
Sodium (mg)	372	Vitamin B_{12} (µg)	1.2
Potassium (mg)	589	Vitamin C (mg)	47

SPINACH-CHEESE FRITTATA DINNER

Menu	*Suggested Serving Sizes*
Tomato soup	¾ cup
Crackers	2
Spinach-Cheese Frittata*	⅙ of recipe
Three-bean salad	½ cup
Skim milk	1 cup
Molasses cookie	1

*Recipe provided

SPINACH-CHEESE FRITTATA (Serves 6)

⅓ cup chopped onions
1 tablespoon margarine
3 eggs
1 package (10½ ounces) chopped spinach, thawed and drained
12 ounces low-fat cottage cheese
1 tablespoon flour
½ teaspoon thyme
1 tomato, sliced
¼ cup fine bread crumbs
¼ cup Parmesan cheese

Directions

1. In a 10-inch, ovenproof skillet, melt margarine and sauté onion until limp.
2. In mixing bowl, beat eggs; then add drained spinach, cottage cheese, flour, and thyme.
3. Pour spinach mixture into skillet and stir with onions.
4. Place skillet into oven and bake at 350 degrees for 35 minutes.
5. Add sliced tomatoes to top; sprinkle with bread crumbs and Parmesan cheese.
6. Turn oven to broil, and broil 1 to 2 minutes until brown.

Composition of Recipe

Serving size: ⅙ of recipe

Calories	155	Zinc (mg)	1.0
Protein (g)	14	Iron (mg)	2.2
Total Fat (g)	7	Vitamin A (IU)	4560
Carbohydrate (g)	9	Thiamin (mg)	0.1
Cholesterol (mg)	136	Riboflavin (mg)	0.3
Fiber (g)	1.3	Niacin (mg)	0.7
Calcium (mg)	165	Vitamin B_6 (mg)	0.3
Magnesium (mg)	47	Folacin (free) (µg)	59
Sodium (mg)	382	Vitamin B_{12} (µg)	0.7
Potassium (mg)	321	Vitamin C (mg)	17

Appetizers

MIDDLE EASTERN HUMMUS (Makes 2 cups)

½ cup sesame seeds
1 large onion, chopped
3 garlic cloves, minced
1 tablespoon olive oil
1 can (16 ounces) chickpeas or garbanzo beans, drained and rinsed
1½ teaspoons lemon juice
1 tablespoon soy sauce
¼ cup tahini paste
Pita bread

Directions

1. Place sesame seeds on a cookie sheet; toast at 300 degrees for 10 to 15 minutes, or until lightly browned.
2. In a skillet, sauté onion and garlic in olive oil until limp.
3. Place toasted sesame seeds in a blender or food processor, and blend into a paste.
4. Add sautéed mixture and remaining ingredients and blend until smooth.
5. Serve by dipping pieces of pita bread into the hummus.

Composition

Serving size: 2 tablespoons hummus and 1 pita bread

Calories	176	Zinc (mg)	1.6
Protein (g)	6	Iron (mg)	1.8
Total Fat (g)	6	Vitamin A (IU)	10
Carbohydrate (g)	23	Thiamin (mg)	0.1
Cholesterol (mg)	1	Riboflavin (mg)	0.1
Fiber (g)	5.4	Niacin (mg)	1.2
Calcium (mg)	51	Vitamin B_6 (mg)	0.1
Magnesium (mg)	27	Folacin (free) (µg)	11
Sodium (mg)	219	Vitamin B_{12} (µg)	0
Potassium (mg)	149	Vitamin C (mg)	1

SOY CHICKEN WINGS (Makes 16 appetizers)

⅔ cup sugar
⅔ cup water
½ cup reduced-sodium soy sauce
16 raw chicken wings
¼ teaspoon black pepper
½ teaspoon garlic powder

Directions

1. In a blender, combine sugar, water, and soy sauce.
2. Marinate wings in this mixture for 6 hours or overnight in the refrigerator.
3. Remove wings and place into a 9" × 13" baking dish. Season wings with pepper and garlic powder.
4. Bake, covered, for 1½ hours at 375 degrees.
5. Uncover and bake 30 minutes longer until wings are brown.

Composition

Serving size: 1 chicken wing

Calories	79	Zinc (mg)	0.4
Protein (g)	7	Iron (mg)	0.7
Total Fat (g)	2	Vitamin A (IU)	12
Carbohydrate (g)	9	Thiamin (mg)	0
Cholesterol (mg)	17	Riboflavin (mg)	0.1
Fiber (g)	0	Niacin (mg)	1.5
Calcium (mg)	11	Vitamin B_6 (mg)	0.1
Magnesium (mg)	36	Folacin (free) (μg)	3
Sodium (mg)	410	Vitamin B_{12} (μg)	0.1
Potassium (mg)	77	Vitamin C (mg)	0

TANGY PORKBALLS (Makes 48 small meatballs)

1 pound fresh-ground low-fat pork
3 bread slices, torn
2 tablespoons brown sugar
½ teaspoon dry mustard
1 tablespoon soy sauce
¼ cup water
Sauce for dipping:
⅔ cup apricot jam
3 tablespoons horseradish

Directions

1. Mix ground pork and torn bread crumbs, and shape into 1-inch balls.
2. Spray heavy skillet with vegetable spray; brown meatballs over medium heat.
3. Remove meatballs from skillet and set aside; remove fat from skillet.
4. In the skillet, combine sugar, mustard, soy sauce, and water; bring to a boil.
5. Return meatballs to skillet and cook, turning frequently; cook until liquid is reduced.
6. Serve meatballs hot with mixture of apricot jam and horseradish for dipping sauce.

Composition

Serving size: 2 meatballs and sauce

Calories	90	Zinc (mg)	0.4
Protein (g)	4	Iron (mg)	0.4
Total Fat (g)	4	Vitamin A (IU)	1
Carbohydrate (g)	9	Thiamin (mg)	0.1
Cholesterol (mg)	14	Riboflavin (mg)	0.1
Fiber (g)	0.1	Niacin (mg)	0.9
Calcium (mg)	7	Vitamin B_6 (mg)	0.1
Magnesium (mg)	8	Folacin (free) (µg)	2
Sodium (mg)	83	Vitamin B_{12} (µg)	0.1
Potassium (mg)	72	Vitamin C (mg)	0

TINY TOSTADAS (Makes 24 appetizers)

1 can refried beans
¼ cup taco sauce
24 round tortilla chips
½ cup shredded cheddar cheese
10 to 12 cherry tomatoes, each cut into 3 to 4 slices

Directions

1. Mix refried beans with taco sauce.
2. Spread 1 teaspoon of mixture on each chip.
3. Top each with small amount of shredded cheese.
4. Place 6 to 8 tostadas on a microwave-safe plate lined with a paper towel.
5. Microwave, uncovered, at medium power for 1 to 3 minutes.
6. Top each with tomato slice.

Note: This recipe is best when *not* made ahead of time.

Composition

Serving size:	1 appetizer		
Calories	48	Zinc (mg)	0.2
Protein (g)	2	Iron (mg)	0.3
Total Fat (g)	3	Vitamin A (IU)	236
Carbohydrate (g)	5	Thiamin (mg)	0
Cholesterol (mg)	2	Riboflavin (mg)	0
Fiber (g)	0.8	Niacin (mg)	0.3
Calcium (mg)	27	Vitamin B_6 (mg)	0
Magnesium (mg)	69	Folacin (free) (µg)	7
Sodium (mg)	91	Vitamin B_{12} (µg)	0
Potassium (mg)	84	Vitamin C (mg)	4

Salads

CREAMY LO-CAL COLESLAW (Serves 8)

4 cups shredded raw cabbage
½ cup red or green pepper, chopped
¼ cup milk
2 tablespoons cider vinegar
½ cup low-calorie mayonnaise
2 tablespoons sugar

Directions

1. In a large bowl, combine cabbage and chopped pepper.
2. In a small bowl, blend milk, vinegar, mayonnaise, and sugar.
3. Pour dressing over the cabbage mixture; stir to mix.

Composition

Serving size:	½ cup		
Calories	81	Zinc (mg)	0.3
Protein (g)	1	Iron (mg)	0.3
Total Fat (g)	5	Vitamin A (IU)	152
Carbohydrate (g)	7	Thiamin (mg)	0
Cholesterol (mg)	2	Riboflavin (mg)	0
Fiber (g)	0.7	Niacin (mg)	0.2
Calcium (mg)	35	Vitamin B_6 (mg)	0.1
Magnesium (mg)	12	Folacin (free) (µg)	16
Sodium (mg)	116	Vitamin B_{12} (µg)	0
Potassium (mg)	158	Vitamin C (mg)	37

CUCUMBERS WITH ROSEMARY AND THYME (Serves 8)

4 cups cucumber slices (2 cucumbers, unpared and scored)
½ small onion, thinly sliced
½ teaspoon salt
1½ tablespoons water
1½ tablespoons olive oil
2 tablespoons red wine vinegar
1 tablespoon Dijon-style mustard
1 teaspoon sugar
1 teaspoon dried rosemary
1 teaspoon thyme leaves, crushed
⅛ teaspoon black pepper

Directions

1. Place cucumbers and onion in a small bowl with lid.
2. Combine all remaining ingredients; pour over cucumbers and onions.
3. Refrigerate. Toss to coat every few hours.

Composition

Serving size: ⅛ of recipe

Calories	41	Zinc (mg)	0.1
Protein (g)	1	Iron (mg)	0.4
Total Fat (g)	3	Vitamin A (IU)	2
Carbohydrate (g)	3	Thiamin (mg)	0
Cholesterol (mg)	0	Riboflavin (mg)	0
Fiber (g)	0.4	Niacin (mg)	0.2
Calcium (mg)	20	Vitamin B_6 (mg)	0
Magnesium (mg)	7	Folacin (free) (µg)	9
Sodium (mg)	162	Vitamin B_{12} (µg)	0
Potassium (mg)	131	Vitamin C (mg)	8

ORANGE-ONION SALAD (Serves 4)

2 tablespoons oil
2 teaspoons tarragon vinegar
1 teaspoon sugar
⅛ teaspoon salt
3 drops hot sauce
⅛ teaspoon pepper
2 large oranges
¼ red onion, cut into rings
Lettuce leaves

Directions

1. In a small bowl or jar, combine oil, vinegar, sugar, salt, hot sauce, and pepper. Stir or shake thoroughly and set aside.
2. Line salad plates with lettuce leaves. Peel orange with a knife, removing membrane. Cut each orange into 6 round slices.
3. Arrange orange slices and onion rings on lettuce leaves.
4. Before serving, pour oil and vinegar mixture over salad.

Composition

Serving size:	¼ of recipe		
Calories	114	Zinc (mg)	0.4
Protein (g)	2	Iron (mg)	0.7
Total Fat (g)	7	Vitamin A (IU)	336
Carbohydrate (g)	13	Thiamin (mg)	0.1
Cholesterol (mg)	0	Riboflavin (mg)	0.1
Fiber (g)	1.9	Niacin (mg)	0.5
Calcium (mg)	46	Vitamin B_6 (mg)	0.1
Magnesium (mg)	22	Folacin (free) (µg)	4.2
Sodium (mg)	75	Vitamin B_{12} (µg)	0
Potassium (mg)	254	Vitamin C (mg)	47

Soups

Greek Lemon Soup (Serves 6)

2 cans (10¾ ounces each) condensed chicken broth
2 cans (10¾ ounces each) water
½ cup uncooked rice
2 egg yolks
¼ cup lemon juice
1 peeled lemon, cut into paper-thin slices, if desired
Snipped fresh chives, if desired

Directions

1. Heat chicken broth in large saucepan over medium heat to boiling; stir in rice.
2. Cook uncovered, stirring occasionally, until rice is soft, about 15 minutes.
3. In a small bowl, whisk egg yolks and lemon juice until light and lemon colored.
4. Whisk 1 cup of hot broth gradually into egg yolk mixture.
5. Remove saucepan from heat; slowly stir egg yolk mixture into broth.
6. Garnish soup with lemon slices and chopped chives.

Composition

Serving size: ⅙ of recipe

Calories	113	Zinc (mg)	0.6
Protein (g)	7	Iron (mg)	1.2
Total Fat (g)	3	Vitamin A (IU)	170
Carbohydrate (g)	15	Thiamin (mg)	0.1
Cholesterol (mg)	85	Riboflavin (mg)	0.1
Fiber (g)	2.6	Niacin (mg)	2.8
Calcium (mg)	20	Vitamin B_6 (mg)	0.1
Magnesium (mg)	7	Folacin (free) (µg)	9
Sodium (mg)	832	Vitamin B_{12} (µg)	0.2
Potassium (mg)	206	Vitamin C (mg)	5

SPRING VEGETABLE SOUP (Serves 8)

1 tablespoon olive oil
1 onion, thinly sliced
2 cloves garlic, finely chopped
1 small eggplant, peeled and cubed (about 1½ cups)
1 medium-sized zucchini, sliced
½ green pepper, seeded and diced
2 fresh tomatoes, chopped
5 cups water
1¼ teaspoons basil
½ teaspoon coriander
¾ teaspoon oregano
1 teaspoon salt
¼ teaspoon pepper
½ cup small shell macaroni, uncooked

Directions

1. Heat olive oil in a heavy kettle; sauté the onions and garlic until tender but not browned.
2. Add the eggplant, zucchini, and green pepper; cook, stirring over medium heat until lightly browned, about 8 to 10 minutes.
3. Add remaining ingredients except macaroni. Bring to a boil, cover, and simmer 10 minutes or until vegetables are barely tender.
4. Add macaroni, cover, and allow to rest for 10 minutes.

Composition

Serving size:	1 cup		
Calories	80	Zinc (mg)	0.3
Protein (g)	3	Iron (mg)	1.1
Total Fat (g)	2	Vitamin A (IU)	451
Carbohydrate (g)	14	Thiamin (mg)	0.1
Cholesterol (mg)	0	Riboflavin (mg)	0.1
Fiber (g)	1.2	Niacin (mg)	1.1
Calcium (mg)	32	Vitamin B_6 (mg)	0.1
Magnesium (mg)	23	Folacin (free) (µg)	10
Sodium (mg)	271	Vitamin B_{12} (µg)	0
Potassium (mg)	254	Vitamin C (mg)	25

TURKEY BARLEY SOUP (Serves 8)

1 turkey carcass
8 cups water
⅓ cup barley
1½ cups chopped onion
¼ cup chopped fresh parsley
1 bay leaf
1 teaspoon poultry seasoning
1 cup sliced carrots
½ cup sliced celery
1 can (16 ounces) tomatoes
1 teaspoon salt-free Creole seasoning
1 teaspoon salt

Directions

1. Place turkey carcass in large kettle or stockpot and cover with water. Bring to a boil, then simmer for 1½ hours, covered. Turn carcass, if necessary, during cooking.
2. Remove carcass. Strip meat from bones and add to broth.
3. Add barley; bring to a boil and simmer 15 minutes.
4. Add remaining ingredients and seasonings. Cook until vegetables are tender, about 15 minutes.

Composition

Serving size:	1 cup		
Calories	70	Zinc (mg)	0.7
Protein (g)	8	Iron (mg)	2.3
Total Fat (g)	1	Vitamin A (IU)	2650
Carbohydrate (g)	9	Thiamin (mg)	0.1
Cholesterol (mg)	13	Riboflavin (mg)	0.1
Fiber (g)	1.3	Niacin (mg)	3.1
Calcium (mg)	45	Vitamin B_6 (mg)	0.2
Magnesium (mg)	25	Folacin (free) (µg)	18
Sodium (mg)	304	Vitamin B_{12} (µg)	0.1
Potassium (mg)	347	Vitamin C (mg)	21

Entrees

SLIMMING SEAFOOD SALAD (Serves 3)

1 pound skinned fish fillets, fresh or frozen
1 cup boiling water
2 tablespoons lemon juice
½ small onion, thinly sliced
½ teaspoon salt
2 peppercorns or dash of pepper
1 medium sprig of parsley
½ bay leaf
Salad greens
Tomato, cucumber, and celery
Low-calorie dressing

Directions

1. Place fillets into a lightly oiled 10-inch skillet. Add remaining ingredients except salad greens and fresh vegetables.
2. Cover and simmer 5 to 10 minutes or just until fish flakes easily when tested with fork. Carefully remove, drain, and place in a covered dish. Chill in refrigerator.
3. Arrange salad greens in bowl or plate with chilled poached fish and fresh vegetables.
4. Serve with 1 to 2 tablespoons of low-calorie dressing.

Composition

Serving size: ⅓ of recipe

Calories	145	Zinc (mg)	0.9
Protein (g)	22	Iron (mg)	1.8
Total Fat (g)	2	Vitamin A (IU)	870
Carbohydrate (g)	11	Thiamin (mg)	0.1
Cholesterol (mg)	35	Riboflavin (mg)	0.1
Fiber (g)	1.2	Niacin (mg)	2.3
Calcium (mg)	93	Vitamin B_6 (mg)	0.2
Magnesium (mg)	50	Folacin (free) (µg)	33
Sodium (mg)	717	Vitamin B_{12} (µg)	0.8
Potassium (mg)	708	Vitamin C (mg)	29

VERMICELLI SALAD (Serves 6)

1 package (7 ounces) vermicelli coils (about 3 cups cooked)
½ cup chopped red onion
½ green pepper, chopped
1 tablespoon chopped parsley
1 teaspoon celery seed
½ teaspoon oregano
½ teaspoon chopped chives
¼ cup low-calorie mayonnaise
¼ cup plain low-fat yogurt
12 ounces cooked shrimp or crab meat, marinated in
　½ cup lemon juice (optional)

Directions

1. Cook vermicelli in boiling water, stirring constantly; drain and blanch with cold water.
2. Add onion, green pepper, parsley, celery seed, chives, oregano, and Italian dressing.
3. Combine mayonnaise with yogurt and add to salad mixture.

Composition

Serving size:　⅙ of recipe

Calories	218	Zinc (mg)	1.6
Protein (g)	18	Iron (mg)	3.0
Total Fat (g)	5	Vitamin A (IU)	193
Carbohydrate (g)	25	Thiamin (mg)	0.1
Cholesterol (mg)	81	Riboflavin (mg)	0.1
Fiber (g)	0.6	Niacin (mg)	2.1
Calcium (mg)	106	Vitamin B_6 (mg)	0.1
Magnesium (mg)	53	Folacin (free) (µg)	10
Sodium (mg)	244	Vitamin B_{12} (µg)	0.5
Potassium (mg)	232	Vitamin C (mg)	28

SHANGHAI CHICKEN SALAD (Serves 4)

2 cups cooked skinless chicken, diced and refrigerated until cool
2 tablespoons tahini sauce
2 tablespoons reduced-sodium soy sauce
2 teaspoons white vinegar
⅛ teaspoon red pepper (cayenne)
1 green onion, chopped
1 tablespoon fresh cilantro (coriander), chopped
1 tablespoon water
½ head lettuce, shredded
2 tablespoons peanuts, chopped

Directions

1. In a small bowl, combine tahini sauce, soy sauce, and vinegar.
2. Blend in red pepper, green onion, and cilantro. Whisk until thoroughly blended. Mix in water.
3. Gently combine chicken with sauce.
4. Mound lettuce on a platter or individual plates; arrange chicken salad on lettuce and sprinkle with chopped peanuts.

Composition

Serving size: ¼ of recipe

Calories	200	Zinc (mg)	2.0
Protein (g)	23	Iron (mg)	1.6
Total Fat (g)	10	Vitamin A (IU)	243
Carbohydrate (g)	4	Thiamin (mg)	0.1
Cholesterol (mg)	64	Riboflavin (mg)	0.2
Fiber (g)	1.0	Niacin (mg)	7.8
Calcium (mg)	34	Vitamin B_6 (mg)	0.4
Magnesium (mg)	48	Folacin (free) (µg)	23
Sodium (mg)	419	Vitamin B_{12} (µg)	0.2
Potassium (mg)	305	Vitamin C (mg)	3

TURKEY PASTA SALAD (Serves 5)

2 cups smoked cooked turkey, cut in ½-inch cubes
4 cups cooked pasta (8 ounces dry)
¼ cup chopped green or red pepper
¼ cup chopped green onion
1 cup cherry tomatoes, cut in half
⅓ cup plain low-fat yogurt
⅓ cup buttermilk
3 tablespoons olive oil
3 tablespoons red wine vinegar
1 tablespoon lemon juice
½ teaspoon celery seed
4 drops hot sauce
⅛ teaspoon black pepper
¼ teaspoon garlic powder
Lettuce leaves

Directions

1. In a large bowl, combine cubed turkey, cooked pasta, green pepper, green onion, and tomatoes.
2. For dressing, combine all the remaining ingredients in a container, cover tightly, and shake until thoroughly mixed.
3. Pour dressing over turkey mixture and stir gently to blend.
4. Serve turkey pasta on lettuce leaves.

Composition

Serving size: ⅕ of recipe

Calories	363	Zinc (mg)	1.9
Protein (g)	26	Iron (mg)	2.2
Total Fat (g)	13	Vitamin A (IU)	685
Carbohydrate (g)	38	Thiamin (mg)	0.2
Cholesterol (mg)	45	Riboflavin (mg)	0.2
Fiber (g)	0.8	Niacin (mg)	8.4
Calcium (mg)	65	Vitamin B_6 (mg)	0.3
Magnesium (mg)	48	Folacin (free) (µg)	20
Sodium (mg)	78	Vitamin B_{12} (µg)	0.4
Potassium (mg)	526	Vitamin C (mg)	25

CREOLE RED SNAPPER (Serves 8)

2 pounds fresh red snapper fillets, cut into 3-inch pieces
1 package (10 ounces) okra
1 can (29 ounces) tomatoes, crushed
1 large onion, chopped
¼ teaspoon Tabasco™ sauce
½ teaspoon filé powder
½ teaspoon salt
2 tablespoons olive oil

Directions

1. In a casserole dish, mix olive oil and chopped onion. Add dash of Tabasco sauce.
2. Layer with ½ package of okra, then add layer of 1 pound of fish; cover with ½ can of tomatoes.
3. Sprinkle tomatoes with ½ teaspoon filé; repeat layering of okra, fish, and tomatoes. On top layer of tomatoes, sprinkle chopped onion.
4. Bake at 350 degrees for 45 minutes.

Suggestion: Serve in large soup bowl with crusty bread and Tabasco sauce.

Composition

Serving size: ⅛ of recipe

Calories	199	Zinc (mg)	1.5
Protein (g)	30	Iron (mg)	1.9
Total Fat (g)	5	Vitamin A (IU)	1020
Carbohydrate (g)	8	Thiamin (mg)	0.5
Cholesterol (mg)	76	Riboflavin (mg)	0.1
Fiber (g)	1.9	Niacin (mg)	5
Calcium (mg)	74	Vitamin B_6 (mg)	1.1
Magnesium (mg)	70	Folacin (free) (µg)	38
Sodium (mg)	232	Vitamin B_{12} (µg)	1.2
Potassium (mg)	767	Vitamin C (mg)	32

CREOLE SHRIMP CASSEROLE (Serves 4)

8 ounces fresh mushrooms, sliced
1 tablespoon margarine
1 cup shrimp, cooked and cleaned
1 cup cooked rice
½ cup diced green pepper
½ cup chopped onion
¼ cup chopped celery
¼ cup chopped red pepper
1 tomato, finely chopped
¼ teaspoon salt
¼ teaspoon chili powder
¼ teaspoon garlic powder
¾ teaspoon thyme
1 teaspoon filé powder
1 teaspoon basil
1 tomato, thinly sliced

Directions

1. In a skillet, heat margarine and sauté mushrooms until tender.
2. In a large bowl, combine cooked rice, green pepper, onion, celery, red pepper, chopped tomato, and all the seasonings. Add the sautéed mushrooms and mix.
3. Place into a 2-quart microwave-safe casserole and cover with wax paper.
4. Microwave on high for 6 minutes; stir, then microwave another 6 minutes.
5. Stir in cooked shrimp. Top with thinly sliced tomato and cover.
6. Microwave an additional 3 minutes on high.

Composition

Serving size: ¼ of recipe

Calories	166	Zinc (mg)	1.2
Protein (g)	12	Iron (mg)	2.9
Total Fat (g)	4	Vitamin A (IU)	933
Carbohydrate (g)	24	Thiamin (mg)	0.2
Cholesterol (mg)	44	Riboflavin (mg)	0.4
Fiber (g)	4.8	Niacin (mg)	4.2

Calcium (mg)	72	Vitamin B$_6$ (mg)	0.3
Magnesium (mg)	50	Folacin (free) (µg)	31
Sodium (mg)	483	Vitamin B$_{12}$ (µg)	0.2
Potassium (mg)	570	Vitamin C (mg)	55

MICROWAVE FISH FILLETS AMANDINE (Serves 6)

⅓ cup slivered almonds
2 tablespoons margarine
1½ pounds fish fillets
½ teaspoon seasoned salt
1½ tablespoons fresh lemon juice
6 lemon wedges
1 teaspoon seasoned pepper

Directions

1. In microwave oven, toast slivered almonds for 5 to 7 minutes.
2. Melt margarine and blend with seasoned salt and seasoned pepper.
3. Lightly cover fillets with margarine and arrange around the outside of a 2-quart glass dish.
4. Sprinkle fillets with lemon juice and cover dish with wax paper.
5. Microwave for 6 to 8 minutes, rotating dish ¼ turn halfway through the cooking time.
6. Let fillets rest for 5 minutes. Top with toasted almonds and serve with lemon wedges.

Composition

Serving size:	⅙ of recipe		
Calories	206	Zinc (mg)	0.7
Protein (g)	23	Iron (mg)	1
Total Fat (g)	12	Vitamin A (IU)	304
Carbohydrate (g)	2	Thiamin (mg)	0.1
Cholesterol (mg)	40	Riboflavin (mg)	0.1
Fiber (g)	0.2	Niacin (mg)	2.4
Calcium (mg)	39	Vitamin B$_6$ (mg)	0.2
Magnesium (mg)	40	Folacin (free) (µg)	9
Sodium (mg)	234	Vitamin B$_{12}$ (µg)	0.6
Potassium (mg)	360	Vitamin C (mg)	2

RED SNAPPER SUPREME (Serves 4)

1¼ pounds red snapper steaks
2 tablespoons margarine
1 tablespoon fresh parsley
¼ teaspoon basil
½ carrot, minced
1 celery stalk, minced
1 cup white or rosé wine
¼ teaspoon salt
¼ teaspoon pepper
Lemon slices

Directions

1. Melt margarine in baking dish.
2. Arrange fish in dish and cover with parsley, carrots, and celery. Sprinkle basil over top and pour wine overall.
3. Bake uncovered at 350 degrees for 20 to 25 minutes.
4. Arrange snapper on hot platter, and pour sauce over fish. Garnish with lemon slices. Serve immediately.

Microwave Directions

Use microwave-safe baking dish; cover fish and vegetables; microwave on high for 6 to 8 minutes, turning dish once; let rest 2 to 3 minutes before serving.

Composition

Serving size:	¼ of recipe		
Calories	231	Zinc (mg)	1.5
Protein (g)	28	Iron (mg)	1.5
Total Fat (g)	7	Vitamin A (IU)	1340
Carbohydrate (g)	4	Thiamin (mg)	0.2
Cholesterol (mg)	76	Riboflavin (mg)	0
Fiber (g)	0.3	Niacin (mg)	4.1
Calcium (mg)	40	Vitamin B_6 (mg)	1
Magnesium (mg)	49	Folacin (free) (µg)	16
Sodium (mg)	324	Vitamin B_{12} (µg)	1.2
Potassium (mg)	578	Vitamin C (mg)	4

SOLE FILLET WITH SHRIMP SAUCE (Serves 6)

2 packages (12 ounces each) frozen sole fillets, partially thawed
¼ teaspoon pepper
2 tablespoons finely chopped onion
¾ cup dry white wine
2 tablespoons margarine
1½ tablespoons flour
1 cup skim milk
5 ounces frozen, medium-size cooked shrimp, thawed
3 tablespoons chopped fresh parsley

Directions

1. Separate sole fillets; arrange in single layer in lightly greased oven-to-table baking dish (9" × 13").
2. Sprinkle with pepper and onion. Pour wine over fish.
3. Bake uncovered at 325 degrees for 10 to 15 minutes, until fish flakes evenly.
4. While fish is baking, melt margarine in saucepan. Blend in flour and stir to form smooth paste. Gradually add milk, stirring constantly until sauce is thick and smooth, about 5 minutes.
5. When fish is done, pour fish juices into a saucepan and heat over medium heat until juices are reduced to ⅓ cup. Stir into white sauce.
6. Add thawed cooked shrimp to white sauce.
7. Spoon sauce over fish and garnish with parsley.

Composition

Serving size:	⅙ of recipe		
Calories	188	Zinc (mg)	1.3
Protein (g)	24	Iron (mg)	1.9
Total Fat (g)	5	Vitamin A (IU)	375
Carbohydrate (g)	5	Thiamin (mg)	0.1
Cholesterol (mg)	63	Riboflavin (mg)	0.1
Fiber (g)	0.3	Niacin (mg)	2
Calcium (mg)	137	Vitamin B_6 (mg)	0.2
Magnesium (mg)	47	Folacin (free) (µg)	11
Sodium (mg)	319	Vitamin B_{12} (µg)	1
Potassium (mg)	473	Vitamin C (mg)	5

ARMENIAN SHISH KABOBS (Serves 6)

2 pounds boneless lamb, cut into 1-inch cubes
½ teaspoon salt
¼ teaspoon pepper
½ teaspoon celery salt
½ teaspoon paprika
1 teaspoon Worcestershire sauce
2 garlic cloves, crushed
½ teaspoon thyme
¼ cup fresh lemon juice
1 cup plain low-fat yogurt
3 lemons, cut into quarters
6 long skewers

Directions

1. Combine all ingredients except lemon quarters.
2. Place in a resealable, plastic food bag. Refrigerate overnight or 24 hours.
3. Before broiling, thread a lemon quarter on each of the 6 skewers; then thread on the cubes of marinated lamb. End each skewer with a lemon quarter.
4. Broil 3 to 4 inches from heat source for 5 to 6 minutes; turn, then broil additional 5 minutes. (Can also be grilled over charcoal for about 20 minutes or until lamb is tender but still pink inside.)

Note: The yogurt makes basting unnecessary, but kabobs may be basted with any barbecue sauce during the last 5 minutes for more color and flavor.

Composition

Serving size:	⅙ of recipe		
Calories	275	Zinc (mg)	5.5
Protein (g)	36	Iron (mg)	4
Total Fat (g)	10	Vitamin A (IU)	156
Carbohydrate (g)	6	Thiamin (mg)	0.2
Cholesterol (mg)	90	Riboflavin (mg)	0.5
Fiber (g)	0.1	Niacin (mg)	8

Calcium (mg)	67	Vitamin B$_6$ (mg)	0.3
Magnesium (mg)	31	Folacin (free) (µg)	5
Sodium (mg)	291	Vitamin B$_{12}$ (µg)	2.7
Potassium (mg)	544	Vitamin C (mg)	25

SMOKED TURKEY WILD RICE CASSEROLE (Serves 8)

3 cups cooked wild rice
½ pound fresh mushrooms, sliced
4 tablespoons margarine
2 cups diced smoked turkey
1 can (12½ ounces) evaporated skim milk
1½ cups water
2 tablespoons chopped chives
1¾ cups Parmesan cheese, divided

Directions

1. In a large saucepan, melt butter; sauté sliced mushrooms.
2. Add cooked wild rice, diced smoked turkey, evaporated skim milk, water, and chives; mix thoroughly.
3. Pour mixture into a buttered 2½ quart casserole dish. Sprinkle with 1 cup Parmesan cheese.
4. Bake, covered, at 350 degrees for 1 hour.
5. At mealtime, sprinkle each serving with 2 tablespoons Parmesan cheese.

Composition

Serving size: ⅛ of recipe

Calories	319	Zinc (mg)	2.9
Protein (g)	28	Iron (mg)	2
Total Fat (g)	11	Vitamin A (IU)	459
Carbohydrate (g)	27	Thiamin (mg)	0.2
Cholesterol (mg)	49	Riboflavin (mg)	0.6
Fiber (g)	0.8	Niacin (mg)	6.9
Calcium (mg)	407	Vitamin B$_6$ (mg)	0.3
Magnesium (mg)	69	Folacin (free) (µg)	14
Sodium (mg)	299	Vitamin B$_{12}$ (µg)	0.6
Potassium (mg)	476	Vitamin C (mg)	2

STIR-FRY CHICKEN AND BROCCOLI WITH RICE
(Serves 4)

2 chicken breasts, skinned, boned, and thinly sliced
3 tablespoons cornstarch
4 tablespoons low-sodium soy sauce
2 tablespoons peanut oil
½ pound broccoli, broken into small pieces
1 medium onion, sliced or chopped
2 cups fresh bean sprouts
1 cup chicken broth
4 cups hot cooked rice

Directions

1. In a medium bowl, blend cornstarch with soy sauce; add chicken slices and stir until chicken is thoroughly coated. Let stand 15 minutes.
2. Heat oil in wok over high heat. Add chicken and stir-fry until browned.
3. Remove chicken from wok; add broccoli and onion to wok and stir-fry 2 minutes.
4. Add mushrooms, bean sprouts, and chicken to wok; stir in chicken broth.
5. Cover and cook gently for 5 minutes or until vegetables are crisp-tender. Serve with rice.

Composition

Serving size: ¼ of recipe

Calories	506	Zinc (mg)	3.3
Protein (g)	31	Iron (mg)	4.9
Total Fat (g)	13	Vitamin A (IU)	1950
Carbohydrate (g)	69	Thiamin (mg)	0.4
Cholesterol (mg)	59	Riboflavin (mg)	0.4
Fiber (g)	14	Niacin (mg)	8.7
Calcium (mg)	132	Vitamin B_6 (mg)	0.4
Magnesium (mg)	112	Folacin (free) (µg)	27
Sodium (mg)	1536	Vitamin B_{12} (µg)	0.2
Potassium (mg)	666	Vitamin C (mg)	78

TURKEY DIVAN (Serves 4)

1 package (10 ounces) broccoli spears, thawed
½ pound sliced cooked turkey breast
3 tablespoons flour
1 can (10½ ounces) ready-to-serve low-sodium chicken broth
⅓ cup Cheddar cheese, shredded
⅛ teaspoon pepper
⅛ teaspoon salt

Directions

1. Arrange broccoli in bottom of 8" × 8" microwave-safe dish.
2. Layer turkey slices on top of broccoli.
3. Mix flour, salt, and pepper with broth in saucepan or glass measuring cup.
4. Cook, stirring constantly, until thickened; add shredded cheese.
5. Stir until cheese is melted; pour sauce over turkey and broccoli.
6. *Microwave Method:* Cover dish and microwave on high for 9 minutes or until broccoli is done.
   Conventional Method: Bake covered at 375 degrees for 20 to 25 minutes.

Composition

Serving size:	¼ of recipe		
Calories	197	Zinc (mg)	1.9
Protein (g)	27	Iron (mg)	1.7
Total Fat (g)	7	Vitamin A (IU)	1790
Carbohydrate (g)	8	Thiamin (mg)	0.1
Cholesterol (mg)	53	Riboflavin (mg)	0.3
Fiber (g)	2.8	Niacin (mg)	8.4
Calcium (mg)	141	Vitamin B_6 (mg)	0.3
Magnesium (mg)	32	Folacin (free) (µg)	20
Sodium (mg)	572	Vitamin B_{12} (µg)	0.3
Potassium (mg)	528	Vitamin C (mg)	58

LINGUINE WITH TOMATOES AND ZUCCHINI (Serves 6)

4 ounces linguine, cooked and drained (about 2 cups)
1 tablespoon margarine
⅓ cup chopped onion
1 green pepper, seeded and cut into strips
2½ cups sliced zucchini
4 medium tomatoes, peeled, seeded, and cut into strips
¼ cup chopped parsley
¼ cup freshly grated Parmesan cheese
2 ounces low-fat cheese

Directions

1. Melt margarine in skillet and sauté onion for about 5 minutes. Add green pepper and cook a few minutes more.
2. Combine with all remaining ingredients, reserving 2 tablespoons Parmesan cheese for top.
3. Place in greased 2-quart casserole, and sprinkle with remaining Parmesan cheese.
4. Bake covered at 350 degrees for 30 to 40 minutes, or until cheese is bubbling. Do not overcook.

Composition

Serving size:	⅙ of recipe		
Calories	169	Zinc (mg)	0.9
Protein (g)	10	Iron (mg)	2.0
Total Fat (g)	5	Vitamin A (IU)	2130
Carbohydrate (g)	26	Thiamin (mg)	0.2
Cholesterol (mg)	6	Riboflavin (mg)	0.2
Fiber (g)	2.6	Niacin (mg)	2.6
Calcium (mg)	169	Vitamin B_6 (mg)	0.3
Magnesium (mg)	53	Folacin (free) (µg)	40
Sodium (mg)	276	Vitamin B_{12} (µg)	0.1
Potassium (mg)	659	Vitamin C (mg)	83

Vegetables

THREE-CHEESE SCALLOPED POTATOES (Serves 6)

4 large baking potatoes, peeled and cut into slices
⅛ teaspoon dried thyme
2 ounces crumbled blue cheese
2 ounces shredded Monterey Jack cheese
Salt and pepper
1 can (12 ounces) evaporated skim milk
1 teaspoon cornstarch
¼ cup Parmesan cheese

Directions

1. Place potato slices in a saucepan. Add thyme and cover with boiling water.
2. Bring to a boil, cover, lower heat, and simmer 3 minutes. Do not overcook.
3. Draining thoroughly and carefully; layer half the potato slices on bottom of greased, shallow baking dish.
4. Blend blue cheese and shredded Monterey Jack cheese to form a paste.
5. Spread paste over the potato slices in baking pan; sprinkle with salt and pepper.
6. Layer remaining potato slices on top.
7. Dissolve cornstarch in milk, then pour over layered potatoes.
8. Sprinkle with Parmesan cheese.
9. Bake at 350 degrees for 1 hour, or until top is golden brown, potatoes are tender, and the liquid has been absorbed.

Composition

Serving size:	⅙ of recipe		
Calories	182	Zinc (mg)	1.1
Protein (g)	10	Iron (mg)	0.7
Total Fat (g)	6	Vitamin A (IU)	227
Carbohydrate (g)	22	Thiamin (mg)	0.1
Cholesterol (mg)	33	Riboflavin (mg)	0.3
Fiber (g)	0.9	Niacin (mg)	1.4

Calcium (mg)	259	Vitamin B_6 (mg)	0.4
Magnesium (mg)	45	Folacin (free) (μg)	16
Sodium (mg)	221	Vitamin B_{12} (μg)	0.3
Potassium (mg)	497	Vitamin C (mg)	16

MARINATED CARROTS (Serves 10)

2 pounds carrots, scraped and cut into chunks
1 large sliced onion
1 green pepper, cut into slices
1 can (10½ ounces) low-sodium tomato soup
½ cup sugar
¼ cup oil
½ teaspoon pepper
6 tablespoons vinegar
½ teaspoon dillweed

Directions

1. Cook carrots in water until tender; drain.
2. Add sliced onion and green pepper to cooked carrots.
3. In saucepan, combine soup (do not dilute) and remaining ingredients; heat until sugar is dissolved.
4. Pour mixture over carrots, onion, and pepper, and cover. Refrigerate.

Note: If desired, onion and pepper may be omitted.

Composition

Serving size: ⅒ of recipe

Calories	149	Zinc (mg)	0.5
Protein (g)	2	Iron (mg)	0.1
Total Fat (g)	6	Vitamin A (IU)	8710
Carbohydrate (g)	24	Thiamin (mg)	0.1
Cholesterol (mg)	1	Riboflavin (mg)	0.1
Fiber (g)	1.7	Niacin (mg)	0.7
Calcium (mg)	38	Vitamin B_6 (mg)	0.2
Magnesium (mg)	25	Folacin (free) (μg)	14
Sodium (mg)	277	Vitamin B_{12} (μg)	0
Potassium (mg)	383	Vitamin C (mg)	29

ORIENTAL ZUCCHINI (Serves 6)

1 pound zucchini (3 to 4 small)
1 tablespoon reduced-sodium soy sauce
½ teaspoon salt
¼ teaspoon pepper
Vegetable oil spray

Directions

1. Wash zucchini and slice ⅛-inch thick.
2. Lightly spray skillet with vegetable oil spray; add sliced zucchini and cook about 2 minutes.
3. Season with soy sauce, salt, and pepper. Serve hot.

Composition

Serving size: ⅙ of recipe

Calories	12	Zinc (mg)	0.1
Protein (g)	1	Iron (mg)	0.5
Total Fat (g)	0	Vitamin A (IU)	227
Carbohydrate (g)	2	Thiamin (mg)	0
Cholesterol (mg)	0	Riboflavin (mg)	0.1
Fiber (g)	0.5	Niacin (mg)	0.6
Calcium (mg)	22	Vitamin B_6 (mg)	0.1
Magnesium (mg)	17	Folacin (free) (μg)	1
Sodium (mg)	223	Vitamin B_{12} (μg)	0
Potassium (mg)	119	Vitamin C (mg)	7

RED CABBAGE AND APPLES (Serves 4)

4 cups shredded red cabbage
3 tablespoons water
2 medium-sized cooking apples, pared, cored, and sliced
1 tablespoon margarine
1 teaspoon flour
2 tablespoons brown sugar
2 tablespoons vinegar
1 teaspoon salt
⅛ teaspoon pepper

Directions

1. Place shredded cabbage, sliced apples, and water in saucepan.
2. Cook, covered, over medium heat for about 10 minutes.
3. Combine remaining ingredients, add to cabbage and apples, and heat thoroughly.

Microwave Directions

1. Place shredded cabbage, sliced apples, and water in 2½ quart casserole. Cover and microwave for 5 to 6 minutes.
2. Stir, then microwave for 5 to 6 more minutes until apples are tender.
3. Combine remaining ingredients, add to cabbage and apples, and microwave for 1 minute.
4. Let stand, covered, for about 2 minutes before serving.

Composition

Serving size: ¼ of recipe

Calories	119	Zinc (mg)	0.5
Protein (g)	2	Iron (mg)	0.9
Total Fat (g)	4	Vitamin A (IU)	299
Carbohydrate (g)	23	Thiamin (mg)	0.1
Cholesterol (mg)	0	Riboflavin (mg)	0.1
Fiber (g)	2.7	Niacin (mg)	0.4
Calcium (mg)	66	Vitamin B_6 (mg)	0.2
Magnesium (mg)	23	Folacin (free) (μg)	31
Sodium (mg)	595	Vitamin B_{12} (μg)	0
Potassium (mg)	345	Vitamin C (mg)	53

Breads

BANANA BRAN MUFFINS (Makes 12 muffins)

3 tablespoons margarine
6 tablespoons sugar
2 eggs
1½ cups whole-bran cereal
⅓ cup buttermilk
⅔ cup whole wheat flour
½ teaspoon salt
1 teaspoon baking soda
¼ teaspoon allspice
2 ripe bananas, mashed

Directions

1. Cream margarine and sugar; beat in eggs, one at a time.
2. Add cereal and buttermilk.
3. Blend in flour, salt, soda, and allspice.
4. Fold in mashed bananas.
5. Spoon into 12 muffin cups, filling each ¾ full.
6. Bake at 375 degrees for 15 minutes.
Serve with honey.

Composition

Serving size:	1 muffin		
Calories	129	Zinc (mg)	1.7
Protein (g)	4	Iron (mg)	2.1
Total Fat (g)	4	Vitamin A (IU)	653
Carbohydrate (g)	23	Thiamin (mg)	0.2
Cholesterol (mg)	42	Riboflavin (mg)	0.2
Fiber (g)	3.9	Niacin (mg)	2.2
Calcium (mg)	27	Vitamin B_6 (mg)	0.3
Magnesium (mg)	57	Folacin (free) (µg)	46
Sodium (mg)	328	Vitamin B_{12} (µg)	0.1
Potassium (mg)	244	Vitamin C (mg)	7

BREAKFAST BRAN MUFFINS (Makes 30 muffins)

1 cup boiling water
1 cup Nabisco 100% All-Bran
½ cup plus 1 tablespoon vegetable shortening
1¼ cups sugar
2 eggs, beaten
2 cups buttermilk
2 cups Kellogg's All-Bran cereal
2½ cups whole-wheat flour
2½ teaspoons baking soda
½ teaspoon salt

Directions

1. In a separate bowl, pour boiling water over the Nabisco 100% All-Bran.
2. In a large mixing bowl, cream the shortening and sugar; add the beaten eggs and buttermilk.
3. Add Kellogg's All-Bran, flour, baking soda, and salt, and mix.
4. Fold in the soaked Nabisco bran.
   (*Note:* At this point, the batter may be refrigerated in a tightly covered container for up to 6 weeks. If desired, spoon out into greased muffin tins before breakfast and bake.)
5. Fill greased muffin tins about ¾ full. Bake at 400 degrees for 15 to 18 minutes.

Composition

Serving size:	1 muffin		
Calories	128	Zinc (mg)	1.4
Protein (g)	3	Iron (mg)	1.7
Total Fat (g)	4	Vitamin A (IU)	373
Carbohydrate (g)	22	Thiamin (mg)	0.2
Cholesterol (mg)	17	Riboflavin (mg)	0.2
Fiber (g)	3.4	Niacin (mg)	1.8
Calcium (mg)	33	Vitamin B_6 (mg)	0.2
Magnesium (mg)	44	Folacin (free) (μg)	34
Sodium (mg)	221	Vitamin B_{12} (μg)	0.1
Potassium (mg)	164	Vitamin C (mg)	4

RAISIN SCONES (Makes 8 scones)

1¾ cups flour
2 teaspoons baking powder
1 tablespoon sugar
½ teaspoon salt
¼ cup shortening
1 egg, beaten
½ cup milk
⅓ cup raisins
1 teaspoon sugar

Directions

1. Combine the flour, baking powder, 1 tablespoon sugar, and salt.
2. Cut the shortening into the mixture until it is coarse.
3. Add the beaten egg, milk, and raisins to the flour mixture. Combine with a few strokes until the dough leaves the side of the bowl. Handle as little as possible.
4. Place dough on a lightly greased baking pan; pat (with lightly floured hands) into a round shape about ¾ inch thick. Sprinkle with 1 teaspoon sugar, and cut into 8 wedges.
5. Bake at 425 degrees for 12 to 15 minutes. Serve at once with jam.

Composition

Serving size:	1 scone		
Calories	192	Zinc (mg)	0.4
Protein (g)	4	Iron (mg)	1.1
Total Fat (g)	7	Vitamin A (IU)	61
Carbohydrate (g)	28	Thiamin (mg)	0.1
Cholesterol (mg)	34	Riboflavin (mg)	0.1
Fiber (g)	1.2	Niacin (mg)	0.9
Calcium (mg)	44	Vitamin B_6 (mg)	0
Magnesium (mg)	11	Folacin (free) (μg)	9
Sodium (mg)	262	Vitamin B_{12} (μg)	0.1
Potassium (mg)	102	Vitamin C (mg)	0

Whole-Wheat Nut Bread (Makes about 22 slices)

1 cup flour
2 cups whole-wheat flour
½ cup sugar
1 teaspoon salt
1½ tablespoons baking powder
3 eggs, beaten
3 tablespoons oil
1½ cups milk
1 cup chopped nuts

Directions

1. Combine flours, sugar, salt, and baking powder. Mix to blend.
2. Make a "well" in center of the flour mixture, and add beaten eggs, oil, and milk.
3. Stir gently until the mixture is blended, but allow lumps to remain.
4. Stir in chopped nuts.
5. Pour batter into a greased loaf pan (8½" × 4½"). Bake at 350 degrees for 55 to 60 minutes. After cooling, remove from bread pan and cut into slices.

Composition

Serving size:	1 slice		
Calories	151	Zinc (mg)	0.6
Protein (g)	5	Iron (mg)	0.8
Total Fat (g)	7	Vitamin A (IU)	65
Carbohydrate (g)	19	Thiamin (mg)	0.1
Cholesterol (mg)	37	Riboflavin (mg)	0.1
Fiber (g)	1.6	Niacin (mg)	1.8
Calcium (mg)	47	Vitamin B_6 (mg)	0.1
Magnesium (mg)	24	Folacin (free) (µg)	10
Sodium (mg)	419	Vitamin B_{12} (µg)	0.1
Potassium (mg)	111	Vitamin C (mg)	0

Beverages

BANANA BREAKFAST SHAKE (Makes 1 serving)

1 banana
¼ cup orange juice
¼ cup plain low-fat yogurt
1 teaspoon orange marmalade
¼ teaspoon cinnamon
1 teaspoon non-fat dry milk

Directions

Blend all ingredients in a blender or food processor.

Composition

Serving size: Full recipe

Calories	192	Zinc (mg)	0.9
Protein (g)	6	Iron (mg)	1.3
Total Fat (g)	1	Vitamin A (IU)	447
Carbohydrate (g)	42	Thiamin (mg)	0.2
Cholesterol (mg)	4	Riboflavin (mg)	0.3
Fiber (g)	1.9	Niacin (mg)	1.2
Calcium (mg)	161	Vitamin B_6 (mg)	0.7
Magnesium (mg)	75	Folacin (free) (µg)	34
Sodium (mg)	56	Vitamin B_{12} (µg)	0.4
Potassium (mg)	746	Vitamin C (mg)	43

HOT CRANBERRY PUNCH (Makes 10 servings)

1 can (16 ounces) jellied cranberry sauce
3 tablespoons light brown sugar
¼ teaspoon ground cinnamon
¼ teaspoon ground allspice
⅛ teaspoon ground cloves
⅛ teaspoon ground nutmeg
2 cups water
2 cups unsweetened pineapple juice
⅛ teaspoon butter flavoring

Directions

1. In large saucepan, crush the cranberry sauce with a fork.
2. Mix with brown sugar, cinnamon, allspice, cloves, and nutmeg.
3. Add water and pineapple juice. Cover and simmer 2 hours.
4. Just before serving, add the butter flavoring and ladle into mugs.

Composition

Serving size:	5 ounces		
Calories	110	Zinc (mg)	0.1
Protein (g)	0	Iron (mg)	0.4
Total Fat (g)	0	Vitamin A (IU)	15
Carbohydrate (g)	28	Thiamin (mg)	0
Cholesterol (mg)	0	Riboflavin (mg)	0
Fiber (g)	0.3	Niacin (mg)	0.1
Calcium (mg)	16	Vitamin B_6 (mg)	0.1
Magnesium (mg)	7	Folacin (free) (µg)	1
Sodium (mg)	28	Vitamin B_{12} (µg)	0
Potassium (mg)	104	Vitamin C (mg)	7

PEACHY DRINK (Makes 12 servings)

1 package (16 ounces) frozen peach slices, partially thawed
1 can (6 ounces) frozen orange juice concentrate, partially thawed
1 pint (2 cups) frozen nonfat vanilla yogurt, softened
3½ cups low calorie ginger ale, chilled

Directions

1. In a blender or food processor, combine peaches, orange juice concentrate, softened ice cream, and half the ginger ale. Cover.
2. Blend at medium-low speed until smooth; add rest of ginger ale.
3. To serve, pour mixture into beverage glasses. If desired, serve after dinner as a dessert.

Composition

Serving size:	5 ounces		
Calories	75	Zinc (mg)	0.3
Protein (g)	2	Iron (mg)	0.3
Total Fat (g)	0	Vitamin A (IU)	550
Carbohydrate (g)	16	Thiamin (mg)	0.1
Cholesterol (mg)	0	Riboflavin (mg)	0.1
Fiber (g)	0.5	Niacin (mg)	0.6
Calcium (mg)	50	Vitamin B_6 (mg)	0
Magnesium (mg)	14	Folacin (free) (µg)	2
Sodium (mg)	12	Vitamin B_{12} (µg)	0
Potassium (mg)	179	Vitamin C (mg)	31

STRAWBERRY BREAKFAST SHAKE (Makes 1 serving)

½ cup strawberries
¼ cup orange juice
¼ cup plain low-fat yogurt
1 teaspoon orange marmalade
¼ teaspoon ginger
1 teaspoon non-fat dry milk

Directions

Blend all ingredients in a blender or food processor.

Composition

Serving size:	Full recipe		
Calories	119	Zinc (mg)	0.7
Protein (g)	5	Iron (mg)	1
Total Fat (g)	1	Vitamin A (IU)	241
Carbohydrate (g)	23	Thiamin (mg)	0.1
Cholesterol (mg)	4	Riboflavin (mg)	0.2
Fiber (g)	1.5	Niacin (mg)	0.8
Calcium (mg)	160	Vitamin B_6 (mg)	0.1
Magnesium (mg)	29	Folacin (free) (µg)	20
Sodium (mg)	56	Vitamin B_{12} (µg)	0.4
Potassium (mg)	433	Vitamin C (mg)	78

Desserts

APPLE BROWN BETTY (Makes 6 servings)

7 slices dry bread, cubed (2 cups)
4 tablespoons melted margarine
5 cups tart apples (about 3 Granny Smith applies), pared, cored, and sliced
½ cup brown sugar
1½ tablespoon lemon juice
1 teaspoon grated lemon peel
½ teaspoon cinnamon
⅔ cup hot water

Directions

1. Mix bread cubes and margarine in small bowl.
2. Combine apples, brown sugar, lemon juice and peel, and cinnamon in large bowl; toss well.
3. Spread ⅓ of bread mixture in bottom of greased 2-quart baking dish. Top with half of apple mixture. Repeat layers.
4. Top with remaining bread mixture. Pour water over all.
5. Bake covered at 350 degrees for 30 minutes; remove cover. Bake until apples are tender and top is golden brown and crisp, about 30 minutes. Cool slightly.

Composition

Serving size:	⅙ of recipe		
Calories	273	Zinc (mg)	0.3
Protein (g)	3	Iron (mg)	1.7
Total Fat (g)	9	Vitamin A (IU)	385
Carbohydrate (g)	46	Thiamin (mg)	0.1
Cholesterol (mg)	1	Riboflavin (mg)	0.1
Fiber (g)	3	Niacin (mg)	0.8
Calcium (mg)	50	Vitamin B_6 (mg)	0
Magnesium (mg)	21	Folacin (free) (µg)	7
Sodium (mg)	258	Vitamin B_{12} (µg)	0
Potassium (mg)	196	Vitamin C (mg)	6

BLUEBERRIES AND LEMON SHERBET (Makes 4 servings)

1 pint lemon sherbet
1 pint fresh blueberries, washed
4 sprigs fresh mint (optional)

Directions

1. In tall parfait glasses, place a spoonful of blueberries; add a scoop of lemon sherbet.
2. Continue alternating small scoops of lemon sherbet with fresh blueberries; top with blueberries.
3. If desired, garnish with mint sprig and serve with long-handled spoons.

Composition

Serving size:	¼ of recipe		
Calories	179	Zinc (mg)	0.2
Protein (g)	1	Iron (mg)	0.8
Total Fat (g)	2	Vitamin A (IU)	138
Carbohydrate (g)	41	Thiamin (mg)	0
Cholesterol (mg)	0	Riboflavin (mg)	0.1
Fiber (g)	2.1	Niacin (mg)	0.4
Calcium (mg)	26	Vitamin B_6 (mg)	0.1
Magnesium (mg)	13	Folacin (free) (µg)	5
Sodium (mg)	11	Vitamin B_{12} (µg)	0
Potassium (mg)	81	Vitamin C (mg)	12

FRUIT KABOBS (Makes 8 servings)

½ cup sugar
¼ cup lemon juice
¼ cup water
3 tablespoons orange liqueur
2 cups fresh pineapple chunks
1 can (11 ounces) mandarin oranges, drained
3 medium bananas
1 pint fresh strawberries
16 wooden skewers

Directions

1. Combine sugar, juice, water, and liqueur.
2. Pour marinade over pineapple and oranges; cover and refrigerate overnight.
3. Shortly before serving, cut bananas into thick slices, add to fruit in marinade; stir gently to coat. Drain.
4. Alternate chunks of pineapple, orange, and banana on skewers; place strawberry on end of each skewer.
5. Serve on a plate or stick skewers into whole fresh pineapple.

Variation: Fresh peach or nectarine wedges may be used instead of mandarin oranges. Canned pineapple chunks may be substituted for fresh.

Composition

Serving size:	2 kabobs		
Calories	143	Zinc (mg)	0.3
Protein (g)	1	Iron (mg)	1.0
Total Fat (g)	0	Vitamin A (IU)	246
Carbohydrate (g)	33	Thiamin (mg)	0.1
Cholesterol (mg)	0	Riboflavin (mg)	0.1
Fiber (g)	2.1	Niacin (mg)	0.6
Calcium (mg)	28	Vitamin B_6 (mg)	0.3
Magnesium (mg)	34	Folacin (free) (μg)	20
Sodium (mg)	2	Vitamin B_{12} (μg)	0
Potassium (mg)	325	Vitamin C (mg)	44

OLD ENGLISH TRIFLE (Makes 12 servings)

Custard:
¼ cup sugar
1 cup skim milk
4 teaspoons cornstarch
1 teaspoon vanilla
1 egg

Cake:
1 12-ounce custard-flavored angel food cake
1 cup sherry

Filling:

1 package (12 ounces) frozen raspberries, thawed
¼ cup raspberry jam
1 package (2.6 ounces) Amarettini Di Saroonna almond-flavored
  macaroons
1 cup whipping cream, whipped
1 can (8 ounces) sliced cling peaches, drained

Directions

1. In saucepan, mix sugar and cornstarch; add milk. Bring to a boil. Remove from heat and cool 5 minutes. Add vanilla and egg, and beat thoroughly with a whisk.
2. Cut cake vertically into 2 rings. Crumble the inner cake ring into the bottom of a 3-quart trifle bowl or straight-sided bowl. Cut the outer cake ring into long pieces and press them against the sides of the bowl. Pour the sherry over the cake.
3. Reserve 8 macaroons for the topping.
4. Spread the jam over the bottom cake crumbs. Layer half of the raspberries, followed by half of the remaining macaroons. Repeat layering with the rest of the raspberries and macaroons.
5. Pour the custard over the fruit and macaroons. Cover and refrigerate overnight.
6. Top with whipped cream; garnish with peach slices and reserved macaroons.

Composition

Serving size: ½ of recipe

Calories	350	Zinc (mg)	0.5
Protein (g)	6	Iron (mg)	0.7
Total Fat (g)	10	Vitamin A (IU)	433
Carbohydrate (g)	59	Thiamin (mg)	0
Cholesterol (mg)	53	Riboflavin (mg)	0.2
Fiber (g)	1.6	Niacin (mg)	0.5
Calcium (mg)	62	Vitamin B_6 (mg)	0.1
Magnesium (mg)	29	Folacin (free) (µg)	6
Sodium (mg)	108	Vitamin B_{12} (µg)	0.2
Potassium (mg)	214	Vitamin C (mg)	4

PEACH MELBA (Makes 4 servings)

2 large peaches
2 cups fresh raspberries
¼ cup sugar
1 pint vanilla frozen yogurt

Directions

1. Put the peaches in a bowl and cover with boiling water. Leave for no more than 1 minute, then drain and peel them.
2. Cut the peaches in half, carefully remove the pits, and set the fruit aside.
3. Rub the raspberries through a fine sieve into a mixing bowl; sweeten the resulting puree with the sugar.
4. Assemble the dessert by placing 2 scoops of vanilla yogurt in each individual serving glass; place one peach half on top, rounded side up, and spoon over part of the raspberry puree. Serve at once.

Composition

Serving size:	¼ of recipe		
Calories	213	Zinc (mg)	0.7
Protein (g)	5	Iron (mg)	0.8
Total Fat (g)	2	Vitamin A (IU)	730
Carbohydrate (g)	47	Thiamin (mg)	0
Cholesterol (mg)	0	Riboflavin (mg)	0.2
Fiber (g)	4	Niacin (mg)	0.8
Calcium (mg)	130	Vitamin B_6 (mg)	0.1
Magnesium (mg)	38	Folacin (free) (µg)	3
Sodium (mg)	2	Vitamin B_{12} (µg)	0
Potassium (mg)	220	Vitamin C (mg)	13

SPARKLING FRUIT CUP (Makes 10 servings)

1 package (16 ounces) frozen fruit medley
1 pound seedless grapes
2 oranges, peeled and cut up
1 teaspoon grated orange rind
2½ teaspoons honey
1 cup flavored sparkling soda such as black cherry, blueberry, non
    alcoholic ginger beer, or ginger ale

Directions

1. Before cutting up fresh orange, grate 1 teaspoon of rind for
   recipe.
2. In a large bowl, combine fruit medley, grapes, and cut-up
   oranges.
3. Stir in grated orange rind and honey.
4. Just before serving, gently add sparkling soda. Serve in individual fruit cups.

Composition

Serving size: ⅒ of recipe

Calories	107	Zinc (mg)	0.2
Protein (g)	1.6	Iron (mg)	0.4
Total Fat (g)	1	Vitamin A (IU)	244
Carbohydrate (g)	26	Thiamin (mg)	0.1
Cholesterol (mg)	0	Riboflavin (mg)	0
Fiber (g)	1.5	Niacin (mg)	0.4
Calcium (mg)	20	Vitamin B_6 (mg)	0.1
Magnesium (mg)	11	Folacin (free) (µg)	12
Sodium (mg)	5	Vitamin B_{12} (µg)	0
Potassium (mg)	192	Vitamin C (mg)	52

⌒ Appendix B ⌒

Facts About
Vitamins and Minerals

A. Vitamins	Primary Functions	Consequences of Deficiency
Thiamin (vitamin B_1)	• Helps body release energy from carbohydrates ingested • Facilitates growth and maintenance of nerve and muscle tissues • Promotes normal appetite	• Fatigue, weakness • Nerve disorders, mental confusion, apathy • Impaired growth • Swelling • Heart irregularity and failure
Riboflavin (vitamin B_2)	• Helps body capture and use energy released from carbohydrates, proteins, and fats • Aids in cell division • Promotes growth and tissue repair • Promotes normal vision	• Reddened lips, cracks at both corners of the mouth • Fatigue
Niacin (vitamin B_3)	• Helps body capture and use energy released from carbohydrates, proteins, and fats • Assists in the manufacture of body fats • Helps maintain normal nervous system functions	• Skin disorders • Nervous and mental disorders • Diarrhea, indigestion • Fatigue

Consequences of Overdose	Primary Food Sources	Highlights and Notes
• None known. High intakes of thiamin are rapidly excreted by the kidneys.	• Grains and grain products (cereal, rice, pasta, bread) • Pork and ham, liver • Milk, cheese, yogurt • Dried beans and nuts	• There is no "e" on the end of thiamin! • Deficiency rare in the U.S. • Enriched grains and cereals prevent thiamin deficiency.
• None known. High doses are rapidly excreted by the kidneys.	• Milk, yogurt, cheese • Grains and grain products (cereals, rice, pasta, bread) • Liver, poultry, fish • Eggs	• Destroyed by exposure to light
• Flushing, headache, cramps, rapid heartbeat with doses above 1.5 grams per day	• Meats (all types) • Grains and grain products (cereals, rice, pasta, bread) • Dried beans and nuts • Milk, cheese, yogurt	• Niacin has a precursor—tryptophan. Tryptophan, an amino acid, is converted to niacin by the body. Much of our niacin intake comes from tryptophan.

	Primary Functions	Consequences of Deficiency
Vitamin B$_6$ (pyridoxine)	• Needed for reactions that build proteins and protein tissues • Assists in the conversion of tryptophan to niacin • Needed for normal red blood cell formation • Promotes normal functioning of the nervous system	• Irritability, depression • Convulsions, twitching • Muscular weakness • Dermatitis near the eyes • Anemia • Kidney stones
Folate (folacin, folic acid)	• Needed for reactions that utilize amino acids (the building blocks of protein) for protein tissue formation • Promotes the normal formation of red blood cells	• Anemia • Diarrhea • Red, sore tongue • Neural tube defects, low birth weight (in pregnancy) • Cervical cancer (possibly)
Vitamin B$_{12}$ (cyanocobalamin)	• Helps maintain nerve tissues • Aids in reactions that build up protein tissues • Needed for normal red blood cell development	• Neurological disorders (nervousness, tingling sensations, brain degeneration) • Anemia • Fatigue

Consequences of Overdose	Primary Food Sources	Highlights and Notes
• Bone pain, loss of feeling in fingers and toes, muscular weakness, numbness, loss of balance (mimicking multiple sclerosis) • Overdose reported for does of 100 mg or more taken for six months or longer	• Oatmeal, fortified cereals • Bananas, avocados, prunes • Chicken, liver • Dried beans • Meats (all types) • Green and leafy vegetables	• Vitamins go from B_3 to B_6 because B_4 and B_5 were found to be duplicates of vitamins already identified
• No toxicity reported with intakes of 10 mg for up to four months • May cover up signs of vitamin B_{12} deficiency (pernicious anemia)	• Dark, green, leafy vegetables (spinach, collards, romaine) • Broccoli, brussels sprouts • Oranges, bananas • Milk, cheese, yogurt • Liver • Dried beans	• Folate means "foliage." It was first discovered in leafy green vegetables. • This vitamin is easily destroyed by heat.
• None known. Excess vitamin B_{12} is readily excreted by the kidneys or is not absorbed into the bloodstream. • Vitamin B_{12} injections may cause a temporary feeling of heightened energy.	• Animal products: beef, lamb, liver, clams, crab, fish, poultry, eggs • Milk and milk products	• Older people and vegans are at risk for vitamin B_{12} deficiency • Some people become vitamin B_{12} deficient because they are genetically unable to absorb it. • Vitamin B_{12} is found in animal products and microorganisms only.

	Primary Functions	Consequences of Deficiency
Biotin	• Needed for the body's manufacture of fats, proteins, and glycogen	• Depression, fatigue, nausea • Hair loss, dry and scaly skin • Muscular pain
Pantothenic acid (pantothenate)	• Needed for the release of energy from fat and carbohydrates	• Fatigue, sleep disturbances, impaired coordination • Vomiting, nausea
Vitamin C (ascorbic acid)	• Needed for the manufacture of collagen • Helps the body fight infections, repair wounds • Acts as an antioxidant • Enhances iron absorption	• Bleeding and bruising easily due to weakened blood vessels, cartilage, and other tissues containing collagen • Slow recovery from infections and poor wound healing • Fatigue, depression
Vitamin A 1. Retinol	• Needed for the formation and maintenance of mucous membranes, skin, bone • Needed for vision in dim light	• Increased susceptibility to infection, increased severity of infection • Impaired vision • Inability to see in dim light

Consequences of Overdose	Primary Food Sources	Highlights and Notes
• None known. Excesses are rapidly excreted.	• Grain and cereal products • Meats, dried beans, cooked eggs • Vegetables	• Deficiency is extremely rare. May be induced by the overconsumption of raw eggs.
• None known. Excesses are rapidly excreted.	• Many foods contain this vitamin, including meats, grains, vegetables, fruits, and milk.	• Deficiency is very rare.
• Intakes of a gram or more per day can cause nausea, cramps, and diarrhea and may increase the risk of kidney stones. • Temporary deficiency may occur after the use of large doses stops.	• Fruits: oranges, lemons, limes, strawberries, cantaloupe, honeydew melon, grapefruit, kiwi fruit, mango, papaya • Vegetables: broccoli, green and red peppers, collards, tomato, asparagus	• Need increases among smokers (to about 200 mg per day) • Is fragile; easily destroyed by heat and exposure to air
• Vitamin A toxicity leading to death has been reported with the use of "therapeutic" vitamin supplements providing 25,000 IU vitamin A per day over several years. Vitamin A intake from supplements should be kept below 10,000 IU per day. • Nausea, irritability, blurred vision • Increased pressure in the skull • Liver damage • Hair loss, dry skin	• Vitamin A is found in animal products only. • Liver, butter, milk, cheese, eggs	• Symptoms of vitamin A toxicity may mimic those of brain tumors and liver disease. Vitamin A toxicity is sometimes misdiagnosed because of the similarities in symptoms. • 1 μg Retinol equivalent = 5 IU Vitamin A or 6 μg beta-carotene.

	Primary Functions	Consequences of Deficiency
2. Beta-Carotene (a vitamin A precursor or "provitamin")	• Acts as an antioxidant; prevents damage to cell membranes and the contents of cells by repairing damage caused by free radicals	• Deficiency disease related only to lack of vitamin A
Vitamin E (tocopherol)	• Acts as an antioxidant, prevents damage to cell membranes in blood cells, lungs, and other tissues by repairing damage caused by free radicals • Reduces the ability of LDL-cholesterol (the "bad" cholesterol) to form plaque in arteries	• Muscle loss, nerve damage • Anemia • Weakness
Vitamin D (I,25 dihydroxy-cholecalciferol)	• Needed for the absorption of calcium and phosphorus in the gut and in bones	• Weak, deformed bones (children) • Loss of calcium from bones (adults)

Consequences of Overdose	Primary Food Sources	Highlights and Notes
• Appears to be relatively nontoxic • With high intakes and supplemental doses (over 12 mg/day for months), skin may turn yellow-orange. • Possibly related to reversible loss of fertility in women	• Deep orange, yellow, and green vegetables and fruits are often good sources. • Carrots, sweet potatoes, pumpkin, spinach, collards, red peppers, broccoli, cantaloupe, apricots	• The body converts beta-carotene to vitamin A. Other carotenes are also present in food, and some are converted to vitamin A. Beta-carotene and vitamin A perform different roles in the body, however.
• Intakes of up to 800 IU per day are unrelated to toxic side effects	• Oils and fats • Salad dressings, mayonnaise, margarine, shortening, butter • Whole grains, wheat germ • Leafy, green vegetables • Nuts and seeds	• Vitamin E is destroyed by exposure to oxygen and heat. • Oils naturally contain vitamin E. It's there to protect the fat from breakdown due to free radicals. • Supplements do not make people "sexy."
• Mental retardation in young children • Abnormal bone growth and formation • Nausea, diarrhea, irritability, weight loss • Deposition of calcium in organs such as the kidneys, liver, and heart.	• Vitamin D is present in animal products only. • Vitamin D–fortified milk and margarine • Butter • Fish • Eggs • Milk products such as cheese, yogurt, and ice cream are generally not fortified with vitamin D.	• Intakes should not exceed 1,200 IU per day. • Vitamin D is manufactured from cholesterol in cells beneath the surface of the skin upon exposure of the skin to sunlight.

	Primary Functions	Consequences of Deficiency
Vitamin K (phylloquinone, menaquinone)	• Is an essential component of mechanisms that cause blood to clot when bleeding occurs • Aids in the incorporation of calcium into bones	• Bleeding, bruises • Decreased calcium in bones • Deficiency is rare. May be induced by the long-term use (months or more) of antibiotics.

B. Minerals

Calcium	• Component of bones and teeth • Needed for muscle and nerve activity, blood clotting	• Poorly mineralized, weak bones • Stunted growth in children • Convulsions, muscle spasms • Contributes to osteoporosis
Phosphorus	• Component of bones and teeth • Component of certain enzymes and other substances involved in energy formation • Needed to maintain the right acid/base balance of body fluids	• Loss of appetite • Nausea, vomiting • Weakness • Confusion • Loss of calcium from bones

Consequences of Overdose	Primary Food Sources	Highlights and Notes
• Toxicity is only a problem when synthetic forms of vitamin K are taken in excessive amounts. That may cause liver disease.	• Leafy, green vegetables • Grain products	• Vitamin K is produced by bacteria in the gut. Part of our vitamin K supply comes from these bacteria. • Newborns are given a vitamin K injection because they have "sterile" guts and consequently no vitamin K–producing bacteria.
• Drowsiness • Calcium deposits in kidney, liver, and other tissues • Suppression of bone remodeling • Overdose level is 2.5 g or more calcium per day	• Milk and milk products (cheese, yogurt) • Spinach, collard greens • Broccoli • Dried beans	• The average intake of calcium among U.S. women is 74 percent of the RDA. The RDA for men and women aged 19–24 years is 1,200 mg • One in four women in the U.S. develops osteoporosis. • Absorption of calcium is higher from milk and milk products than from plant foods.
• Loss of calcium from bones • Muscle spasms	• Milk and milk products (cheese, yogurt) • Meats • Seeds, nuts • Phosphates added to foods	• Deficiency is generally related to disease processes.

	Primary Functions	Consequences of Deficiency
Magnesium	• Component of bones and teeth • Need for nerve activity • Activates enzymes involved in energy and protein formation	• Stunted growth in children • Weakness • Muscle spasms • Personality changes
Iron	• Transports oxygen as a component of hemoglobin in red blood cells • Component of myo-globin (a muscle pro-tein) • Needed for certain reactions involving energy formation	• Iron deficiency • Iron deficiency anemia • Weakness, fatigue • Pale appearance • Reduced attention span and resistance to infection
Zinc	• Required for the activation of many enzymes involved in the reproduction of proteins • Component of insulin	• Growth failure • Delayed sexual matu-ration • Slow wound healing • Loss of taste and appetite • In pregnancy, low-birth-weight infants and preterm delivery

Consequences of Overdose	Primary Food Sources	Highlights and Notes
• Diarrhea • Dehydration • Impaired nerve activity due to disrupted utilization of calcium	• Plant foods (dried beans, tofu, peanuts, wild rice, bean sprouts, green vegetables)	• Magnesium is primarily found in plant foods where it is attached to chlorophyll. • Average intake among U.S. women is marginally adequate.
• "Iron poisoning" • Hereditary hemochromatosis • Vomiting, abdominal pain • Blue coloration of skin • Shock • Heart failure • Diabetes	• Liver, beef, pork • Dried beans • Iron-fortified cereals • Prunes, apricots, raisins • Spinach	• Cooking foods, especially acid foods like tomatoes, in iron pans dramatically increases the iron content of the foods. • Iron deficiency is the most common nutritional deficiency in the world. • Average iron intake of women in the U.S. is low. • Excessive iron stores in men may be related to the development of heart disease.
• Over 25 mg per day associated with nausea, vomiting, weakness, fatigue, susceptibility to infection, copper deficiency	• Meats (all kinds) • Grains • Nuts • Milk and milk products (cheese, yogurt)	• Like iron, zinc is better absorbed from meats than from plants. • Marginal zinc deficiency may be common, especially in children.

	Primary Functions	Consequences of Deficiency
Iodine	• Component of thyroid hormones that help regulate energy production and growth	• Goiter • Cretinism in newborns (mental retardation, hearing loss, growth failure)
Selenium	• Acts as an antioxidant in conjunction with vitamin E (protects cells from damage due to exposure to oxygen)	• Anemia • Muscle pain and tenderness • "Keshar" disease • Heart failure

Consequences of Overdose	Primary Food Sources	Highlights and Notes
• Over 1 mg per day may produce pimples, goiter, and decreased thyroid function.	• Iodized salt • Milk and milk products • Seaweed, seafood • Bread from commercial bakeries	• Iodine deficiency was a major problem in the U.S. in the 1920s and 1930s. Now intakes are marginally excessive. Deficiency remains a major health problem in some developing countries. • Amount of iodine in plants depends on iodine content of soil. • Most of the iodine in our diet comes from the incidental addition of iodine to foods from the compounds processors use to clean foods.
• Doses of over 2 mg per day associated with "selenosis." Symptoms of selenosis are hair and fingernail loss, weakness, liver damage, irritability, "garlic" or "metallic" breath	• Meats and seafood • Eggs • Grains	• Content in foods depends on amount of selenium in soil, water, and animal feeds. • May play a role in the prevention of some types of cancer.

	Primary Functions	Consequences of Deficiency
Copper	• Component of enzymes involved in the body's utilization of iron and oxygen	• Anemia • Seizures • Nerve and bone abnormalities in children
Fluoride	• Component of bones and teeth (enamel)	• Tooth decay and other dental diseases
Manganese	• Needed for the formation of body fat and bone	• Weight loss • Rash • Nausea and vomiting
Chromium	• Required for the normal utilization of glucose	• Poor blood glucose control • Weight loss
Molybdenum	• Component of enzymes involved in the transfer of oxygen from one molecule to another	• Rapid heartbeat and breathing • Nausea, vomiting • Coma

Consequences of Overdose	Primary Food Sources	Highlights and Notes
• "Wilson's" disease • Vomiting, diarrhea • Tremors • Excessive accumulation of copper in the liver and kidneys • Liver disease	• Oysters, lobster, crab • Liver • Grains • Dried beans • Nuts and seeds	• Toxicity can result from copper pipes and cooking pans. • Average intake in the United States is thought to be marginal.
• "Fluorosis" • Brittle bones • Mottled teeth • Nerve abnormalities	• Fluoridated water and foods and beverages made with it • Tea • Shrimp, crab	• Toothpastes, mouth rinses, and other dental care products may provide fluoride. • Fluoride overdose has been caused by ingestion of fluoridated toothpaste.
• Infertility in men • Disruptions in the nervous system (psychotic symptoms) • Muscle spasms	• Whole grains • Coffee, tea • Dried beans • Nuts	• Toxicity is related to overexposure to manganese dust in miners.
• Kidney and skin damage	• Whole grains • Liver, meat • Beer, wine	• Toxicity usually results from exposure in chrome-making industries.
• Loss of copper from the body • Joint pain • Growth failure • Anemia • Gout	• Dried beans • Grains • Dark green vegetables • Liver • Milk and milk products	• Deficiency is extraordinarily rare.

	Primary Functions	Consequences of Deficiency
Sodium	• Needed to maintain the right acid/base balance in body fluids • Helps maintain an appropriate amount of water in blood and body tissues • Needed for muscle and nerve activity	• Weakness • Apathy • Poor appetite • Muscle cramps • Headache • Swelling
Potassium	• Same as for sodium	• Weakness • Irritability, mental confusion • Irregular heartbeat • Paralysis
Chloride	• Component of hydrochloric acid secreted by the stomach (used in digestion) • Needed to maintain the right acid/base balance of body fluids • Helps maintain an appropriate water balance in the body	• Muscle cramps • Apathy • Poor appetite

Consequences of Overdose	Primary Food Sources	Highlights and Notes
• High blood pressure in susceptible people • Kidney disease • Heart problems	• Foods processed with salt • Cured foods (corned beef, ham, bacon, pickles, sauerkraut) • Table and sea salt	• Very few foods naturally contain much sodium. • Processed foods are the leading source of dietary sodium. • High-sodium diets are associated with the development of hypertension in "salt-sensitive" people.
• Irregular heartbeat, heart attack	• Plant foods (potatoes, squash, lima beans, plantains, bananas, oranges, avocados) • Meats • Milk and milk products	• Content in vegetables is often reduced in processed foods. • Diuretics (water pills) and other antihypertension drugs may deplete potassium. • Salt substitutes often contain potassium.
• Vomiting	• Same as for sodium. (Most of the chloride in our diets comes from salt.)	• Excessive vomiting and diarrhea may cause chloride deficiency.

Sources: Food and Drug Administration (Department of Health and Human Services). Nutrition labeling. Federal Register 1991 November 27; Committee on Diet and Health (Food and Nutrition Board; National Research Council). Diet and Health. Implications for reducing chronic disease risk. Washington, D.C.: National Academy Press, 1989; Present knowledge in nutrition, 6th ed. Washington, D.C.: International Life Sciences Institute, Nutrition Foundation, 1990; and National Academy of Sciences (Institute of Medicine). Recommended Dietary Allowances, 10th ed. Washington, D.C.: Academy of Sciences Press, 1989.

Food Sources of Vitamins and Minerals

A. Vitamins

Vitamin A (Retinol)

Food	Vitamin A (Retinol)	
	Amount	IU*
Meats		
Liver	3 oz	45,400
Crab	½ cup	1,680
Eggs		
Egg	1 medium	590
Milk and Milk Products		
Whole milk	1 cup	330
Skim milk, fortified	1 cup	330
American cheese	1 oz	330
Swiss cheese	1 oz	320
Low-fat milk	1 cup	210
Fats		
Butter	1 tsp	160
Margarine, fortified	1 tsp	160

*5 IU = 1 RE (retinol equivalent)

Beta-Carotene

Food	Beta–Carotene	
	Amount	IU
Vegetables		
Carrots, raw	1 medium	7,900
Sweet potato	½ cup	7,850
Pumpkin	½ cup	7,840
Spinach, cooked	½ cup	7,300
Collard greens, cooked	½ cup	6,030
Winter squash	½ cup	4,200
Ripe peppers	½ cup	2,225
Broccoli	½ cup	1,900
Fruits		
Cantaloupe	¼ whole	5,400
Apricots, canned	½ cup	2,260
Papaya	½ cup	1,595
Watermelon	2 cups	1,265
Peaches, canned	½ cup	1,115
Nectarine	1	1,001

Vitamin D

Food	Vitamin D	
	Amount	IU*
Milk		
Milk, whole, low-fat, or skim	1 cup	100
Fish and Seafood		
Salmon	3 oz	340
Tuna	3 oz	150
Shrimp	3 oz	127
Organ Meats		
Beef liver	3 oz	42
Chicken liver	3 oz	40
Eggs		
Egg yolk	1	27

*40 IU = 1 μg

Vitamin E

Food	Vitamin E	
	Amount	**IU***
Oils		
Oil	1 Tbsp	6.7
Mayonnaise	1 Tbsp	3.4
Margarine	1 Tbsp	2.7
Salad Dressing	1 Tbsp	2.2
Nuts and Seeds		
Sunflower seeds	¼ cup	27.1
Almonds	¼ cup	12.7
Peanuts	¼ cup	4.9
Cashews	¼ cup	0.7
Vegetables		
Sweet potato	½ cup	6.9
Collard greens	½ cup	3.1
Asparagus	½ cup	2.1
Spinach, raw	1 cup	1.5
Grains		
Wheat germ	2 Tbsp	4.2
Bread, whole-wheat	1 slice	2.5
Bread, white	1 slice	1.2
Seafood		
Crab	3 oz	4.5
Shrimp	3 oz	3.7
Fish	3 oz	2.4

*1 IU = 1 mg alpha-tocopherol

Vitamin C

Food	Vitamin C Amount	(mg)
Fruits		
Kiwi fruit	1 or ½ cup	108
Orange juice	6 oz	62
Orange	1	85
Cantaloupe	¼	63
Grapefruit juice	6 oz	57
Grapefruit	½	51
Strawberries	½ cup	48
Cranberry juice cocktail	¾ cup	45
V-8 juice	¾ cup	45
Tomato juice	¾ cup	33
Watermelon	1 cup	31
Grape juice	½ cup	29
Raspberries	½ cup	18
Vegetables		
Green peppers	½ cup	95
Cauliflower, raw	½ cup	75
Broccoli	½ cup	70
Brussels sprouts	½ cup	65
Collard greens	½ cup	48
Cauliflower, cooked	½ cup	30
Potato	1	29
Tomato	½	23

Thiamin

Food	Thiamin	
	Amount	**(mg)**
Meats		
Pork roast	3 oz	0.8
Beef	3 oz	0.4
Ham	3 oz	0.4
Liver	3 oz	0.2
Nuts and Seeds		
Sunflower seeds	¼ cup	0.7
Peanuts	¼ cup	0.1
Almonds	¼ cup	0.1
Grains		
Bran flakes	1 cup	0.6
Macaroni	1 cup	0.2
Rice	1 cup	0.2
Bread	1 slice	0.1
Vegetables		
Peas	½ cup	0.3
Lima beans	½ cup	0.2
Corn	½ cup	0.1
Broccoli	½ cup	0.1
Potato	1	0.1
Fruit		
Orange juice	1 cup	0.2
Orange	1	0.1
Avocado	½	0.1

Riboflavin

Food	Amount	Riboflavin (mg)
Milk and Milk Products		
Milk	1 cup	0.5
Low–fat milk	1 cup	0.5
Yogurt, low–fat	1 cup	0.5
Skim milk	1 cup	0.4
Yogurt	1 cup	0.1
American cheese	1 oz	0.1
Cheddar cheese	1 oz	0.1
Meats		
Liver	3 oz	3.6
Pork chop	3 oz	0.3
Beef	3 oz	0.2
Tuna	½ cup	0.1
Vegetables		
Collard greens	½ cup	0.3
Broccoli	½ cup	0.2
Spinach, cooked	½ cup	0.1
Eggs		
Egg	1	0.2
Grains		
Macaroni	1 cup	0.1
Bread	1 slice	0.1

Niacin

Food	Amount	Niacin (mg)
Meats		
Liver	3 oz	14.0
Tuna	½ cup	10.3
Turkey	3 oz	9.5
Chicken	3 oz	7.9
Salmon	3 oz	6.9
Veal	3 oz	5.2
Beef (round steak)	3 oz	5.1
Pork	3 oz	4.5
Haddock	3 oz	2.7
Scallops	3 oz	1.1
Nuts and Seeds		
Peanuts	1 oz	4.9
Vegetables		
Asparagus	½ cup	1.5
Grains		
Wheat germ	1 oz	1.5
Brown rice	½ cup	1.2
Noodles, enriched	½ cup	1.0
Rice, white, enriched	½ cup	1.0
Bread, enriched	1 slice	0.7
Milk and Milk Products		
Milk	1 cup	1.9
Cottage cheese	½ cup	2.6

Vitamin B₆

Food	Vitamin B₆ Amount	(mg)
Meats		
Liver	3 oz	0.8
Salmon	3 oz	0.7
Other fish	3 oz	0.6
Chicken	3 oz	0.4
Ham	3 oz	0.4
Hamburger	3 oz	0.4
Veal	3 oz	0.4
Pork	3 oz	0.3
Beef	3 oz	0.2
Eggs		
Egg	1	0.3
Legumes		
Split peas	½ cup	0.6
Dried beans, cooked	½ cup	0.4
Fruits		
Banana	1	0.6
Avocado	½	0.4
Watermelon	1 cup	0.3
Vegetables		
Turnip greens	½ cup	0.7
Brussels sprouts	½ cup	0.4
Potato	1	0.2
Sweet potato	½ cup	0.2
Carrots	½ cup	0.2
Peas	½ cup	0.1

Folate

Food	Folate Amount	(µg)
Vegetables		
Asparagus	½ cup	120
Brussels sprouts	½ cup	116
Black-eyed peas	½ cup	102
Spinach, cooked	½ cup	99
Romaine lettuce	1 cup	86
Lima Beans	½ cup	71
Peas	½ cup	70
Collard greens, cooked	½ cup	56
Sweet potato	½ cup	43
Broccoli	½ cup	43
Fruits		
Cantaloupe	¼ whole	100
Orange juice	1 cup	87
Orange	1	59
Grains*		
Breakfast cereals	1 cup	100–400
Oatmeal	½ cup	97
Wheat germ	¼ cup	80
Wild rice	½ cup	37

*Beginning in 1998, refined grain products such as bread, white rice, and pasta are fortified with folic acid and provide approximately 40 µg folate per serving.

Vitamin B$_{12}$

Food	Vitamin B$_{12}$ Amount	(µg)
Meats		
Liver	3 oz	6.8
Trout	3 oz	3.6
Beef	3 oz	2.2
Clams	½ cup	2.0
Crab	3 oz	1.8
Lamb	3 oz	1.8
Tuna	½ cup	1.8
Veal	3 oz	1.7
Hamburger, regular	3 oz	1.5
Milk and Milk Products		
Skim milk	1 cup	1.0
Milk	1 cup	0.9
Yogurt	1 cup	0.8
Cottage cheese	½ cup	0.7
American cheese	1 oz	0.2
Cheddar cheese	1 oz	0.2
Eggs		
Egg	1	0.6

B. Minerals

Calcium

Food	Calcium Amount	(mg)
Milk and Milk Products		
Yogurt, low-fat	1 cup	415
Yogurt with fruit, low-fat	1 cup	315
Skim milk	1 cup	300
Light milk (1%)	1 cup	300
Low-fat milk	1 cup	298
Whole milk	1 cup	288
Swiss cheese	1 oz	270
Cheddar cheese	1 oz	205
Frozen yogurt	1 cup	200
Cream soup	1 cup	186
Pudding	½ cup	185
Ice cream	1 cup	180
Ice milk	1 cup	180
American cheese	1 oz	175
Custard	½ cup	150
Cottage cheese	½ cup	70
Cottage cheese, low-fat	½ cup	69
Vegetables		
Collard greens, cooked	½ cup	110
Spinach, cooked	½ cup	90
Broccoli	½ cup	70
Legumes		
Tofu	½ cup	155
Dried beans, cooked	½ cup	50
Lima beans	½ cup	40

Phosphorus

Food	Phosphorus Amount	(mg)
Milk and Milk Products		
Yogurt	1 cup	327
Skim milk	1 cup	250
Whole milk	1 cup	250
Cottage cheese	½ cup	150
American cheese	1 oz	130
Meats		
Pork	3 oz	275
Hamburger	3 oz	165
Tuna	3 oz	162
Lobster	3 oz	125
Chicken	3 oz	120
Nuts and Seeds		
Sunflower seeds	¼ cup	319
Peanuts	¼ cup	141
Pine nuts	¼ cup	106
Peanut butter	1 Tbsp	61
Grains		
Bran flakes	1 cup	180
Shredded wheat	2 large biscuits	81
Whole-wheat bread	1 slice	52
Vegetables		
Potato	1 medium	101
Corn	½ cup	73
Peas	½ cup	70
French fries	½ cup	61
Broccoli	½ cup	54

Magnesium

Food	Amount	Magnesium (mg)
Legumes		
Lentils, cooked	½ cup	134
Split peas, cooked	½ cup	134
Tofu	½ cup	130
Nuts		
Peanuts	¼ cup	247
Cashews	¼ cup	93
Almonds	¼ cup	80
Grains		
Bran buds	1 cup	240
Wild rice, cooked	½ cup	119
Breakfast cereal, fortified	1 cup	85
Wheat germ	2 Tbsp	45
Vegetables		
Bean sprouts	½ cup	98
Black-eyed peas	½ cup	58
Spinach, cooked	½ cup	48
Lima beans	½ cup	32
Milk and Milk Products		
Milk	1 cup	30
Cheddar cheese	1 oz	8
American cheese	1 oz	6
Meats		
Chicken	3 oz	25
Beef	3 oz	20
Pork	3 oz	20

Iron

Food	Iron Amount	(mg)
Meat and Dried Beans		
Liver	3 oz	7.5
Round steak	3 oz	3.0
Hamburger, lean	3 oz	3.0
Baked beans	½ cup	3.0
Pork	3 oz	2.7
White beans	½ cup	2.7
Soybeans	½ cup	2.5
Pork and beans	½ cup	2.3
Fish	3 oz	1.0
Chicken	3 oz	1.0
Grains		
Breakfast cereal, iron-fortified	1 cup	8.0 (4–18)
Oatmeal, fortified	1 cup	8.0
Bagel	1	1.7
English muffin	1	1.6
Rye bread	1 slice	1.0
Whole-wheat bread	1 slice	0.8
White bread	1 slice	0.6
Fruits		
Prune juice	6 oz	7.0
Apricots, dried	½ cup	2.5
Prunes	5 medium	2.0
Raisins	¼ cup	1.3
Plums	3 medium	1.1
Vegetables		
Spinach, cooked	½ cup	2.3
Lima beans	½ cup	2.2
Black-eyed peas	½ cup	1.7
Peas	½ cup	1.6
Asparagus	½ cup	1.5

Zinc

Food	Zinc	
	Amount	(mg)
Meats		
Liver	3 oz	4.6
Beef	3 oz	4.0
Crab	½ cup	3.5
Lamb	3 oz	3.5
Turkey ham	3 oz	2.5
Pork	3 oz	2.4
Chicken	3 oz	2.0
Legumes		
Dried beans, cooked	½ cup	1.0
Split peas, cooked	½ cup	0.9
Grains		
Breakfast cereal, fortified	1 cup	1.5–4.0
Wheat germ	2 Tbsp	2.4
Brown rice	1 cup	1.2
Oatmeal	1 cup	1.2
Bran flakes	1 cup	1.0
White rice	1 cup	0.8
Nuts and Seeds		
Pecans	¼ cup	2.0
Cashews	¼ cup	1.8
Sunflower seeds	¼ cup	1.7
Peanut butter	2 Tbsp	0.9
Milk and Milk Products		
Cheddar cheese	1 oz	1.1
Whole milk	1 cup	0.9
American cheese	1 oz	0.8

Selenium

Food	Selenium Amount	(mg)
Seafood		
Lobster	3 oz	66
Tuna	3 oz	60
Shrimp	3 oz	54
Oysters	3 oz	48
Fish	3 oz	40
Meats		
Liver	3 oz	56
Ham	3 oz	29
Beef	3 oz	22
Bacon	3 oz	21
Chicken	3 oz	18
Lamb	3 oz	14
Veal	3 oz	10
Eggs		
Egg	1 medium	37

Sodium

Food	Sodium Amount	(mg)
Miscellaneous		
Salt	1 tsp	2,132
Dill pickle	1 (4½ oz)	1,930
Sea salt	1 tsp	1,716
Chicken broth	1 cup	1,571
Ravioli, canned	1 cup	1,065
Spaghetti with sauce, canned	1 cup	955
Baking soda	1 tsp	821
Beef broth	1 cup	782
Gravy	¼ cup	720
Italian dressing	2 Tbsp	720
Pretzels	5 (1 oz)	500
Green olives	5	465
Pizza with cheese	1 wedge	455
Soy sauce	1 tsp	444
Meats		
Corned beef	3 oz	808
Ham	3 oz	800
Fish, canned	3 oz	735
Meatloaf	3 oz	555
Sausage	3 oz	483
Hot dog	1	477
Fish, smoked	3 oz	444

Potassium

Food	Amount	Potassium (mg)
Vegetables		
Potato	1 medium	780
Winter squash	½ cup	327
Tomato	1 medium	300
Celery	1 stalk	270
Carrots	1 medium	245
Broccoli	½ cup	205
Fruits		
Avocado	½ medium	680
Banana	1 medium	440
Orange juice	6 oz	375
Raisins	¼ cup	370
Watermelon	2 cups	315
Prunes	4 large	300
Meats		
Fish	3 oz	500
Hamburger	3 oz	480
Lamb	3 oz	382
Pork	3 oz	335
Chicken	3 oz	208
Grains		
Bran buds	1 cup	1,080
Bran flakes	1 cup	248
Raisin bran	1 cup	242
Wheat flakes	1 cup	96
Milk and Milk Products		
Yogurt	1 cup	531
Skim milk	1 cup	400
Whole milk	1 cup	370
Other		
Salt substitutes	1 tsp	1,300–2,378

Glossary

Abortion   Loss of an embryo or fetus usually within the first three months of pregnancy.

Absorption   The taking up of fluids, gases, and nutrients by the gastrointestinal tract.

Allergy   Unusual or exaggerated sensitivity to a substance that is harmless in similar amounts to most people.

Amino Acids   The chemical building blocks from which proteins are made. Amino acids are classified into two groups: essential and nonessential.

> **Essential**   Amino acids that cannot be produced by the body and must be supplied by the diet. The eight essential amino acids for adults are isoleucine, leucine, lysine, methionine, phenylalanine, theronine, tryptophan, and valine. In addition, histidine and agrinine are required by children for growth.

> **Nonessential**   Amino acids that can be produced by the body provided the diet contains enough nitrogen-containing foods. Nonessential amino acids are alanine, aspartic acid, arginine, citrulline, cystine, glutamic acid, glycine, hydroxyglutamic acid, norleucine, proline, serine, and tyrosine.

Anemia   Reduction in size or number of the red blood cells, of the quantity of hemoglobin, or of both, resulting in decreased capacity of the blood to carry oxygen. The symptoms of anemia are varied and include breathlessness on exertion, easy fatigue, pallor, dizziness, insomnia, and lack of appetite. Anemia may be caused by a deficient intake of nutrients necessary for the formation of blood. Iron, protein, folic acid, vitamin B_{12}, and vitamin C deficiencies interfere with blood formation. Anemia may also be due to blood loss, inherited conditions, and other disorders.

Appetite   The desire for food, founded on learning or memory and related to the agreeable taste, smell, or appearance of food.

Basal Metabolism Energy, or calories, used by the body for maintaining processes such as body temperature, circulation, and muscle tone. Basal metabolism increases during pregnancy, primarily because of increases in body weight, circulation, and protein-tissue formation.

Basic Food Groups Classes of foods listed together under one heading because of their similarities as good sources of certain nutrients. The basic food groups are used in planning and evaluating diets for nutritional adequacy.

Calorie A unit of heat. In nutrition, calorie refers to the amount of heat a food substance will release when completely burned. Approximately 3500 extra calories from food are needed to produce one pound of body fat. Conversely, reducing food intake by 3500 calories below usual intake will cause a weight loss of one pound.

Carbohydrate The class of foods that includes simple sugars and starches. Fiber is a carbohydrate, although it is not digested or absorbed by the body. Carbohydrates are the major sources of calories in most diets.

Cardiac Output The quantity of blood pumped into circulation by the heart per minute. Cardiac output increases substantially during pregnancy.

Cholesterol The chief sterol in the body found in all tissues, especially the brain, nerves, adrenal cortex, and liver. It is also a constituent of bile and serves as a precursor of vitamin D. Cholesterol in the body comes from two sources: dietary cholesterol, chiefly from egg yolk, liver, and meats; and cholesterol made by the liver and other organs. High blood cholesterol levels are related to hardening of the arteries, high blood pressure, stone formation, and other diseases. Blood levels of cholesterol rise substantially during pregnancy.

Constipation Infrequent or difficult bowel movements. Common causes of constipation include a diet low in fiber and fluids, lack of exercise, excessive use of laxatives, and anxiety or worry.

Convenience Foods Foods that have been partially or completely prepared to save time in food preparation.

Diabetic Diet   A diet prescribed for a person with diabetes. This diet follows the pattern of a normal diet for maintenance of good health and normal activity. It is no longer necessary to require a diabetic (who is experiencing no complications from diabetes) to follow detailed dietary regulations and precise food measurements and meal patterns. Except for simple sugars that are rapidly absorbed and can produce high blood-sugar peaks, a diabetic can have more freedom in his or her choice of foods. However, individualization is the rule. The dietary requirements of diabetics differ with the type and extent of insulin received and the amount of activity performed. The most important consideration is adjustment of total caloric intake to attain and maintain desirable body weight. Also important are the proper spacing and regularity of meals, particularly among those receiving insulin, to avoid low blood-sugar levels.

Diarrhea   The frequent passage of loose and watery stools. Severe or prolonged diarrhea can lead to dehydration and mineral losses from the body.

Diet   The foods and beverages a person eats on a regular basis. The diet of most adult Americans includes 200 to 350 different foods and beverages out of approximately 20,000 types of foods and beverages available.

Dietary Counseling   A process of providing individualized professional guidance to assist a person in adjusting his or her daily food consumption to meet health needs.

Diet, Balanced   A diet containing all the required nutrients in proper proportion with respect to one another for optimum nutrition.

Dietetics   The science of the use of foods in health and disease.

Dietitian   One who is professionally qualified by education and experience to provide nutritional care, and apply the science and art of nutrition in helping people of all ages, sick or well, individually or in groups, to meet their nutritional needs. The American Dietetic Association is responsible for qualifications and registration of dietitians in the United States.

Digestion The mechanical and chemical breakdown of food substances into consistent parts. The conversion of food into smaller and simpler units that can be absorbed by the body.

Eclampsia A condition usually occurring during the later half of pregnancy characterized by edema, high blood pressure, proteinuria, and convulsions. The condition is referred to as preeclampsia in the absence of convulsions. Both terms, eclampsia and preeclampsia, are collectively called toxemia of pregnancy.

Edema A condition in which the body tissues contain an excessive amount of fluid. The swelling of body tissues from the excess fluid may be throughout the body or in the legs and ankles, depending upon the seriousness of the condition.

Embryo The developing human organism from conception to eight weeks in the uterus.

"Empty Calorie" Foods A term used to describe foods and beverages that are high in calories and contain small amounts of nutrients. Some nutritionists and mothers have been heard to call such products "junk food."

Energy Capacity to do work. Energy needed by the body for movement and body processes is obtained from food. The energy available from foods is released for use by the body when foods are broken down by enzymes. The amount of energy available from foods is measured in terms of calories.

Energy Balance (Also called calories balance.) The equilibrium between calorie intake and calorie output. When more calories are available from foods eaten than are needed by the body, the surplus is stored as fat. When fewer calories are consumed than needed, the body draws upon the fat stores.

Enrichment The addition of vitamins and minerals (specifically, thiamin, riboflavin, niacin, and iron) to processed cereal and grain products to restore the amount lost in milling and processing.

Estrogen The name given to the female sex hormones produced by the ovary. Estrogens include estrone, estradial, and esterone. Estrogens are responsible for the development of physical sexual characteristics and have a profound influence on reproduction, how the body uses nutrients, and many other processes.

Fetus The body within the uterus from the third month of pregnancy until birth. Before three months, the term embryo is used.

Fiber Substances, primarily carbohydrates, that are found in foods but are not digested by the body. Fiber is needed to promote regular bowel movements. Whole gain breads and cereals, legumes, nuts, seeds, and fruits and vegetables are good sources of dietary fiber.

Food Additive Substances that have been added to food, either intentionally or unintentionally, that are not normally part of the food. Food additives are used to improve the nutritional value, appearance, shelf-life, texture, and flavor of foods. Some additives unintentionally end up in food through processing, production, storage, and packaging. Accidental contaminants, such as mercury or lead, are not considered food additives.

Food Poisoning Toxic condition caused by eating a food contaminated with bacteria.

Fortification Addition of one or more nutrients such as vitamins, minerals, amino acids, and protein concentrates to food so that it contains more nutrients than were originally present. For example, the addition of vitamin A to margarine, vitamin D to milk, lysine to bread, and iodine to salt.

Gastrointestinal Tract Refers to the whole of the digestive tract from the mouth through the stomach, intestines, and anus.

Gestation Pregnancy; the period of fetal development.

Gestational Age The age of a fetus or newborn computed from the first day of the last menstrual period to birth. Most babies are born within a gestational period of thirty-eight to forty-two weeks. Babies that are born unusually small considering the length of pregnancy, or gestation, are classified as small-for-gestational age. Babies that are unusually large for the length of the pregnancy are classified as large-for-gestational age.

Glucose Tolerance Test (GTT) The test that measures the ability of the body to use a certain amount of glucose. It is performed after a twelve-hour fast. The person is given 50 to 100 g of glucose. Blood samples for a glucose analysis are obtained before the glucose is taken and then one-half, one, two, three, and four hours after ingestion. A normal individual shows a rise in blood sugar after about one-half hour after ingestion of glucose, but the blood-sugar level returns to normal after two hours. A person with diabetes shows a much higher rise in blood sugar after one-half hour, which continues to rise even higher after two hours and remains higher than normal after four hours.

Health   State of physical, mental, and emotional well-being, not merely the freedom from disease or the absence of any ailment.

Heartburn   A burning sensation in the esophagus when acidic fluids are forced up from the stomach. It may occur ten to fifteen minutes after eating a big meal, especially if a person lies down after the meal. During pregnancy, heartburn usually results from the pressure of the baby on the stomach.

Hematocrit   A laboratory test that determines the volume of red blood cells in a certain amount of blood. The hematocrit result is used to test for iron deficiency anemia during pregnancy. A hematocrit of less than 33 percent may indicate the development of anemia.

Hemoglobin   The iron-containing substance in red blood cells. Hemoglobin carries the oxygen from the lungs to the tissues. A test for hemoglobin level is usually done several times during pregnancy. A hemoglobin level of less than 11 g percent is suggestive of iron deficiency anemia.

Hemorrhoid   An enlarged bundle of vessels located around the anus.

Heredity   The tendency of a human to reproduce the characteristics of his or her ancestors. Characteristics of heredity are carried in genes located within the sperm and ovum.

Hormone   A chemical substance produced by the body that is carried in the bloodstream to other parts of the body. Each hormone has a specific effect on only those cells and tissues that serve as "targets" for hormonal action.

Hunger   A physical sensation resulting from the lack of food and a sign that food is needed by the body. Hunger is usually accompanied by weakness and an overwhelming desire to eat. It is different from appetite, which is a pleasant sensation based on enjoyment of foods and eating, and not necessarily on the need for food.

Hypertension An increase in blood pressure above normal. Blood pressure varies considerably among individuals. Hypertension often causes dizziness, headaches, poor vision, shortness of breath, chest pain, and poor memory. Blood pressure normally decreases during the early part of pregnancy but returns to pre-pregnancy levels toward the end of pregnancy.

Immunity Resistance to a particular disease. Immunity may be received by the fetus from the mother's blood or may occur as a result of having a disease or receiving a vaccination.

Incidence The number of new cases of a disease or disorder appearing in a set amount of time (usually one year) within a population.

Infant Babies up to one year of age.

Infant Formula A breast milk substitute prepared for infants according to a specific formula.

Infection The transfer of disease from one person to another by a variety of routes.

Lactation Breast-feeding. The production of milk by the breast. The amount of milk a woman produces is affected by her nutritional status, the frequency and length of sucking by the baby, certain drugs (particularly birth-control pills), and hormones.

Lactose Intolerance Failure to digest lactose, a primary component of milk owing to the lack of the enzyme lactose which digests it. Lactose intolerance among infants results in failure to grow and diarrhea if human or cow's milk is given. The condition is extremely rare among infants, particularly breast-fed infants. Adults not used to drinking milk may develop gas pains and diarrhea after drinking a sizable amount of milk. In these cases, small amounts of milk should be taken until the body can produce enough lactose to properly digest it.

Legumes Edible seeds, such as beans, peas, peanuts, and soybeans.

Low Birth-Weight Infant An infant who weighs less than five pounds, eight ounces, or 2500 g at birth.

Malformation A deformity or defective formation of some body part of parts.

Malnutrition A state of poor health with symptoms that can be identified as the result of an inadequate or excessive intake of one or more essential nutrients.

Nutrient A substance needed by the body to perform one or more of the following functions: to provide energy, to build and repair tissues, and to regulate life processes. The body uses about sixty different nutrients from foods. Nutrients are grouped into six categories; proteins, fats, carbohydrates, vitamins, minerals, and water. All nutrients are needed for growth and health. No one nutrient is more important than any other.

Nutrient Deficiency Disease A disease or disorder caused by a dietary deficiency of one or more nutrients. The disease or disorder can be prevented by eating an adequate diet, or in most cases cured by supplying the deficient nutrient or nutrients.

Nutrient Toxicity A disease or disorder caused by taking an excessive amount of certain vitamin and mineral supplements.

Nutrition The science of how the body uses foods and how foods influence health and disease.

Nutritional Status The health condition of a person as influenced by the consumption and utilization of foods.

Nutritionist A dietitian with graduate-level training in nutrition who applies the science of nutrition to improving health, the prevention of disease, and the treatment of disease.

Obesity A condition that exists when a person's weight exceeds by 20 to 30 percent the average weight for persons of the same sex, height, and age.

Overweight A condition that exists when a person's weight exceeds by 10 to 20 percent the average weight for persons of the same sex, height, and age.

Pica The craving and eating of materials not considered food. Common substances craved and consumed include clay, dirt, laundry starch, and ice. Pica may develop during pregnancy and be abandoned after delivery.

Preeclampsia A condition of pregnancy characterized by hypertension, proteinuria, and swelling. The signs of preeclampsia may not be noted until after mid-pregnancy. However, the condition itself begins to develop earlier in pregnancy.

Pregnancy Also called gestation; the condition of having a developing embryo or fetus in the body after the union of an ovum with a spermatozoan. In women the period of pregnancy is about 255 to 280 days. It is divided into three main phases: implantation, the first two weeks of gestation during which the fertilized ovum becomes embedded in the wall of the uterus and the placenta develops; organogenesis, the next ten weeks during which the developing fetal tissue undergoes organ formation; and growth, the remaining eight months, characterized by a rapid growth in organ size and body weight.

Premature A baby born before thirty-seven weeks of gestation. In the past, the term was applied to low birth-weight infants (less than five-and-one-half pounds). The term is now used solely to indicate a shorter-than-average gestational period.

Protein The source of amino acids needed from foods. Protein is a structural component of all tissues. An important function of protein is the manufacture of body tissues such as muscles, bones, nerves, teeth, hair, skin, blood, and organs. All enzymes and some hormones are composed of protein.

Protein Quality An attribute of a protein that depends on the kinds and amounts of amino acids present. In general, plant proteins are lacking or "limiting" in the essential amino acids lysine, methionine, thereonine, and tryptophan. Animal proteins are of high quality, or are said to be complete proteins. A complete protein contains all the essential amino acids in amounts sufficient for growth and life maintenance. An incomplete protein cannot support life or growth. Incomplete sources of protein can be used effectively for growth and repair by combining them with small amounts of complete proteins, or by mixing several plant proteins to obtain a complete assortment of amino acids in the amounts needed for growth and repair.

Proteinuria The presence of protein or amino acids in urine.

Recommended Dietary Allowances The specific term used by the Food and Nutrition Board of the National Research Council of the National Academy of Sciences (NAS/NRC) for recommendations for daily intake of specific nutrients for groups of healthy individuals according to age and sex. The recommended dietary allowances (RDA), designed to be adequate for practically all the population of the United States, allow for a margin of safety.

Satiety   The lack of desire to continue to eat. A feeling of satisfaction after eating.

Starvation   Complete or partial absence from food for varying lengths of time.

Toxicity   A pathological condition that results when harmful substances are ingested or when excessive amounts of normally harmless substances are ingested.

Undernutrition   Inadequate intake of one or more nutrients and/or of calories.

Underweight   The term applied to individuals whose body weights are more than 10 percent below average for individuals of the same age, sex, and height.

Uterus   The womb. A pear-shaped, hollow muscular organ in the female that shelters and nourishes the fetus during pregnancy. Except during pregnancy, the uterus is about three inches long, two inches wide, and one inch thick. It includes the fundus (the upper and broad portion), the body (the central part), and the cervix at the bottom.

Vegans   Individuals who eat only food and food products from plant sources; all animal foods including meat, fish, poultry, milk, eggs, cheese, and seafoods in any form are avoided.

Vegetarians   Those who refrain from eating meat of any kind, but who use milk, milk products, and eggs; these people are more specifically described as ovo-lacto-vegetarians. Those who refrain from eating meat and eggs are called lactovegetarians.

Vulnerability   Susceptible to injury. In nutrition, the phrase vulnerable group refers to infants, children, pregnant or lactating women, and elderly people—groups particularly prone to develop nutritional disorders.

Water Balance   Balance between water input and output. Water intake comes from fluids and beverages, as part of food, or as a product of the breakdown of foods in the body. The channels of water output are through the kidneys (urine), the skin (sweat and insensible perspiration), the lungs (expired air), and the gastrointestinal tract (saliva and feces). Water intake must equal output; a difference results in edema or dehydration, depending on whether intake is greater or less than output. Control of water intake is by thirst. Water output is controlled by hormones. Abnormal losses of water may occur in diarrhea, excessive vomiting, and severe burns.

Weaning The period from the first consistent addition of a semisolid or solid food into the infant diet.

References

Chapter 1

Barker, D. J .P. "Fetal growth and long-term consequences." In J. Boulton, et al. (eds.): *Long–term Consequences of Early Feeding* vol. 36. Philadelphia: Nestec Ltd., Vevey/Lippincott-Ravey Publishers, 1996.

Brown, J. E., and E. S. B. Kahn. "Maternal and nutrition and the outcome of pregnancy: A renaissance in research." *Clinics in Perinatology* (July, 1997).

Godfrey, K. M., and D. J. P. Barker. "Maternal nutrition in relation to fetal and placental growth." *European Journal of Obstetrics, Gynecology and Reproductive Biology* 61:15–22, 1995.

Gonzalez–Cossio T., and H. Delgado. "Functional consequences of maternal malnutrition." *World Review of Nutrition and Dietetics,* 64:139–173, 1981.

Harding, J. E., and B. M. Johnston. "Nutrition and fetal growth." *Reproductive Fertility and Development* 7:539–547, 1995.

Villar, J., and T. G. Cossio. "Nutritional factors associated with low birth weight and short gestational age." *Clinical Nutrition* 5:78–85, 1986.

Chapter 2

Brown, J. E. *Nutrition Now.* St. Paul, Minn.: West Publishing Company, 1995.

The Vegetarian Resource Group, *Vegetarian Journal,* P.O. Box 1463, Baltimore, Md. 21203 (410–366–VEGE).

WWW

Food and Drug Administration provides FDA Consumer Magazine, posts information on biotechnology, food additives, pesticides, and the "bad bug book" on food safety: http://vm.cfsan.fda.gov/list.html

Nutrition and Your Health: Dietary Guidelines for Americans. Download the guidelines from the world wide web. Single copies of the Dietary Guidelines for Americans are available free from the National Maternal and Child Health Clearing House, 2070 Chain Bridge Road, Suite 450, Vienna, VA 22181–2536.

Consumer Nutrition Hotlines

Consumer Nutrition Hotline, National Center for Nutrition and Dietetics, American Dietetic Association: Registered Dietitian referrals and nutrition messages in English and Spanish: 1–800–366–1655.

Chapter 3

Brown, J. E. "Preconceptional nutrition and reproductive outcomes." *Annals of the New York Academy of Sciences* 678:286–292, 1993.

Clark, A. M., et al. "Weight loss results in significant improvement in pregnancy and ovulation rates in anovulatory obese women." *Human Reproduction* 10:2705–2712, 1995.

Guzick, D. F. "Do infertility tests discriminate between fertile and infertile populations?" *Human Reproduction* 10:2008–2009, 1995.

Hatch, E. E., M. B. Bracken. "Associations of delayed conceptions with caffeine consumption." *American Journal of Epidemiology* 138:1082–1092, 1993.

Warren, M. P. "Effects of undernutrition on reproductive function in the human." *Endocrine Reviews* 4:363–377, 1983.

Chapter 4

ACOG Technical Bulletin: "Preconceptional care." *International Journal of Gynecology and Obstetrics* 50:210–217, 1995.

Brown, J. E., and E. S. Kahn. "Maternal nutrition: A renaissance in research." *Clinics in Perinatology* (July 1997).

——— et al. "Predictors of red cell folate level in women attempting pregnancy." *Journal of the American Medical Association* (February 19, 1997).

Enkin, M. W., et al. "Effective care in pregnancy and child birth: A synopsis." *Birth* 22:101–110, 1995.

Gadsby, R., et al. "A prospective study of nausea and vomiting during pregnancy." *British Journal of General Practice* 43:245–248, 1993.

Hinds, T. S., et al. "The effect of caffeine on pregnancy outcome variables." *Nutrition Reviews* 54:203–207, 1996.

"Nutrition During Pregnancy." *ACOG Technical Bulletin* no. 179 (April 1993), *International Journal of Gynecology and Obstetrics* 43:67–74, 1993.

Rosenthal, M. Sara. *The Pregnancy Sourcebook,* 2d ed. Los Angeles: Lowell House, 1997.

Chapter 5

Brown, J. E., and E. S. Kahn. "Maternal nutrition: A renaissance in research." *Clinics in Perinatology* (July 1997).

Institute of Medicine, National Academy of Sciences. *Nutrition During Pregnancy,* Washington, D.C.: National Academy of Sciences Press, 1990.

"Nutrition During Pregnancy." *ACOG Technical Bulletin* no. 179 (April 1993), *International Journal of Gynecology and Obstetrics* 43:67–74, 1993.

Rosso, P. *Nutrition and Metabolism in Pregnancy.* New York: Oxford University Press, 1990.

Chapter 6

Hambidge, M., et al. "Neural tube defects in serum zinc." *British Journal of Obstetrics and Gynecology* 100:746–749, 1993.

Hathcock, J. N. "Safety limits for nutrient intake: Concepts and data requirements." *Nutrition Reviews* 51:278–285, 1993.

Institute of Medicine, National Academy of Sciences. *Nutrition During Pregnancy,* Washington, D.C.: National Academy of Sciences Press, 1990.

Long, P. J. "Rethinking iron supplements in pregnancy." *Journal of Nurse/Midwifery* 40:36–40, 1995.

"Nutrition During Pregnancy." *ACOG Technical Bulletin* no. 179 (April 1993), *International Journal of Gynecology and Obstetrics* 43:67–74, 1993.

Roodenburg, A. J. C. "Iron supplementation during pregnancy." *European Journal of Obstetrics, Gynecology and Reproductive Biology* 61:65–71, 1995.

Rothman, K. J., et al. "Teratogenicity of high vitamin A intake." *New England Journal of Medicine* 333:1369–1373, 1995.

U.S. Preventive Services Task Force. "Routine iron supplementation during pregnancy: Policy statement." *Journal of the American Medical Association* 270:2846–2848, 1993.

Yip, R. "Iron supplementation during pregnancy: Is it effective?" *American Journal of Clinical Nutrition* 63:853–855, 1996.

Chapter 7

Brown, J. E. "Weight gain during pregnancy: What is optimal?" *Clinical Nutrition* 7:181–190, 1988.

Brown J. E., and E. S. B. Kahn. "Maternal and nutrition and the outcome of pregnancy: A renaissance in research." *Clinics in Perinatology* July 1997.

Cogswell, M. E., et al. "Attempted weight loss during pregnancy." *International Journal of Obesity,* 20:373–375, 1996.

Institute of Medicine, National Academy of Sciences. *Nutrition During Pregnancy,* Washington, D.C.: National Academy of Sciences Press, 1990.

Keppel, K. G., and S. M. Taffel. "Pregnancy–related weight gain and retention: Implications of the 1990 Institute of Medicine Guidelines." *American Journal of Public Health,* 83:1100–1103, 1993.

Chapter 8

"Exercise during pregnancy and the postpartum period." *ACOG Technical Bulletin* no. 189:1–4, 1994.

Hatch, M. C., et al. "Maternal exercise during pregnancy, physical fitness, and fetal growth." *American Journal of Epidemiology* 137:1108–1123, 1993.

Spinillo, A., et al. "The effect of work activity in pregnancy on the risk of fetal growth retardation." *Atca Obstetrica et Gynecologica Scandinavica* 75:531–536, 1996.

Sternfeld, B. "Physical activity and pregnancy outcome—Review and rec-ommendations." *Sports Medicine* 23:33–47, 1997.

Zhang, J., and D. A. Sabitz. "Exercise during pregnancy among U.S. women." *Annals of Epidemiology* 6:53–59, 1996.

Chapter 9

Bucher, H. C., et al. "Effect of calcium supplementation on pregnancy–induced hypertension and preeclampsia: A metaanalysis of randomized controlled trials." *Journal of the American Medical Association* 275:111–117, 1996.

Gadsby, R., et al. "A prospective study of nausea and vomiting during preg-nancy." *British Journal of General Practice* 43:245–248, 1993.

Greenberg, L. R., et al. "Gestational diabetes mellitus—Antenatal variables as predictors of postpartum glucose intolerance." *Obstetrics and Gynecology* 86:97–101, 1995.

Institute of Medicine, National Academy of Sciences. *Nutrition During Pregnancy.* Washington, D.C: National Academy of Sciences Press, 1990.

Jovanovic–Peterson, L., and C. M. Peterson. "Exercise and the nutritional management of diabetes during pregnancy." *Obstetrics and Gynecology Clinics of North America* 23:75–86, 1996.

Kesmodel, U., et al. "Marine N–3 fatty acids and calcium intake in relation to pregnancy–induced hypertension, intrauterine growth retardation, and preterm delivery. A case–control study." *Acta Obstetricia et Gynecologica Scandinavica* 76:34–44, 1997.

Kousen, M. "Treatment of nausea and vomiting in pregnancy." *American Family Physician* 48:1279–1283, 1993.

Roodenburg, A. J. C. "Iron supplements during pregnancy." *European Journal of Obstetrics, Gynecology, and Reproductive Biology* 61:65–71, 1995.

Vutyavanich, T., et al. "Pyridoxine for nausea and vomiting of pregnancy: A randomized double-blind, placebo-controlled trial." *American Journal of Obstetrics and Gynecology* 173: 881–884, 1995.

Chapter 10

Brown, J. E., et al. "Prepregnancy weight status, prenatal weight gain, and the outcome of term twin gestations." *American Journal of Obstetrics and Gynecology* 162:182–186, 1990.

Dimperio, D. L. "Nutritional management of multiple pregnancy." *The Perinatal Nutrition Report,* 6–7 (fall 1994).

Institute of Medicine, National Academy of Sciences. *Nutrition During Pregnancy.* Washington, D.C.: National Academy of Sciences Press, 1990.

Lantz, M. E., et al. "Maternal weight gain patterns and birth weight outcome in twin gestation." *Obstetrics and Gynecology* 87:551–556, 1996.

Chapter 11

American Academy of Pediatrics, Committee on Nutrition. "The use of whole cow's milk in infancy." *Pediatrics* (October 1992).

Lambert, E. J., and M. L. Paul. "Infant nutrition." *British Journal of Hospital Medicine* 53:567–70, 1995, and 54:327–330, 1996.

Satter, E. "The feeding relationship: Problems and interventions." *Journal of Pediatrics* 117:5181–5189, 1990.

Story, M., and J. E. Brown . "Do young children instinctively know what to eat? The studies of Clara Davis revisited." *New England Journal of Medicine* 316:103–106, 1987.

Chapter 12

Cunningham, A. S. "Breast-feeding and health." *Journal of Pediatrics* 4:658–659, 1987.

Freed, G. L., et al. "National assessment of physicians' breast-feeding knowledge, attitudes, training, and experience." *Journal of the American Medical Association* 273:472–476, 1995.

Institute of Medicine, National Academy of Sciences. *Nutrition During Lactation.* Washington, D.C.: National Academy Press, 1991.

Rogan, W. G. "Pollutants in breast milk." *Archives of Pediatrics and Adolescent Medicine* 150:981–990, 1996.

Spencer, J. P. "Practical nutrition for the healthy term infant." *American Family Physicians* 54:138–144, 1996.

Strode, M. A., et al. "Effects of short–term caloric restriction on lactational performance of well–nourished women." *ACTA Paediatrica Scandanavia* 75:222–229, 1986.

Wilson, D.C. "Nutrition of the preterm baby." *British Journal of Obstetrics and Gynaecology* 102:854–860, 1995.

Lactation Education and Support

La Leche League International: 1–800–LALECHE.

International Lactation Consultants Association: (708) 260–8874. This number enables you to get an appointment with an internationally board–certified lactation consultant in your area.

WWW

La Leche League International: http://www.prairienet.org/llli/helpform.html.

Maternal and Child Health Net: gopher://mchnet.ichp.ufl.edu:70.

⌒ Index ⌒

⌒ About the Author ⌒

Judith E. Brown, R.D., M.P.H., Ph.D., is a highly regarded expert on maternal nutrition. She is a recipient of the March of Dimes Agnes Higgin's Award for excellence in maternal nutrition research and practice. She is currently chair-elect of the Perinatal Nutrition Practice group of the American Dietetic Association. As a professor of nutrition in the school of public health at the University of Minnesota, Dr. Brown teaches maternal nutrition to nutritionists, midwives, physicians, and medical students and directs the National Maternal Nutrition Intensive Course which is attended yearly by an international audience of health professionals. Dr. Brown has conducted a number of large research studies related to nutrition and reproduction and has published more than 100 scientific articles.